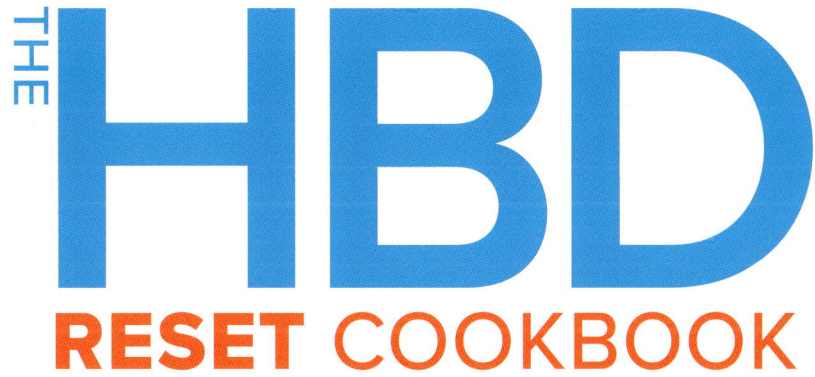

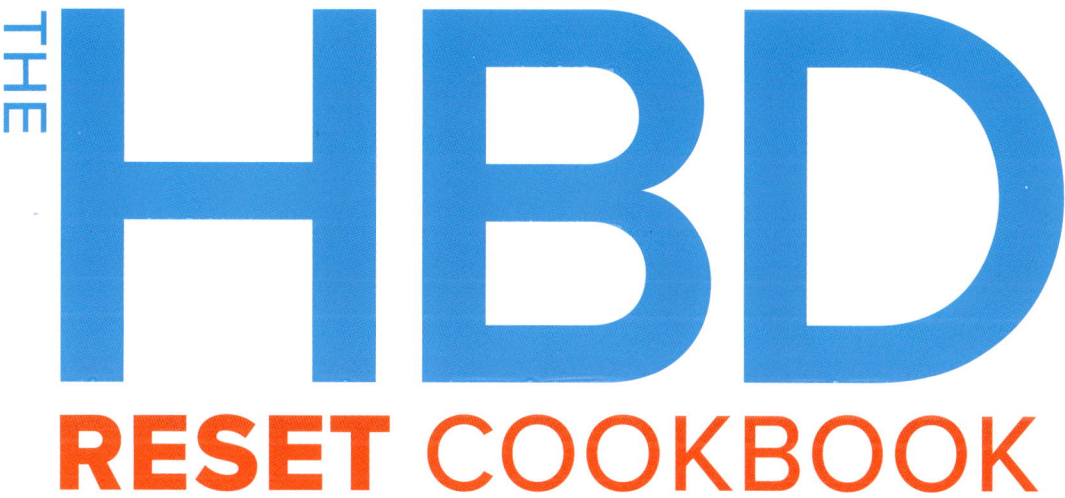

THE HBD
RESET COOKBOOK

The ultimate 16-day bible for
health and perfect weight

Petronella Ravenshear
with recipes by Elisabeth Whiting

Thorsons

Thorsons
An imprint of HarperCollins*Publishers*
1 London Bridge Street
London SE1 9GF

www.harpercollins.co.uk

HarperCollins*Publishers*
Macken House, 39/40 Mayor Street Upper
Dublin 1, D01 C9W8, Ireland

First published by Thorsons 2026

10 9 8 7 6 5 4 3 2 1

Text © Petronella Ravenshear 2026
Recipes © Elisabeth Whiting and Petronella Ravenshear 2026
Photography © Andrew Hayes-Watkins 2026

Petronella Ravenshear asserts the moral right to be identified as the author of this work

A catalogue record of this book is available from the British Library

ISBN 978-0-00-880421-3

Food Stylist: Lizzie Kamenetzky
Prop Stylist: Faye Wears

Printed and bound by GPS in Bosnia & Herzegovina

All rights reserved. No part of this publication may be reproduced, stored in a retrieval system, or transmitted, in any form or by any means, electronic, mechanical, photocopying, recording or otherwise, without the prior written permission of the publishers.

Without limiting the exclusive rights of any author, contributor or the publisher of this publication, any unauthorised use of this publication to train generative artificial intelligence (AI) technologies is expressly prohibited. HarperCollins also exercise their rights under Article 4(3) of the Digital Single Market Directive 2019/790 and expressly reserve this publication from the text and data mining exception.

WHEN USING KITCHEN APPLIANCES PLEASE ALWAYS FOLLOW THE MANUFACTURER'S INSTRUCTIONS

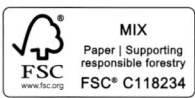

This cookbook is dedicated to you, dear reader, whether this is your first time with HBD or you're returning for your annual Reset. May these recipes tantalise your tastebuds and ensure that the first sixteen days of your HBD adventure are truly delicious.

CONTENTS

INTRODUCTION   9

HBD: The Human Being Diet
– you'll bless the day you started   9

Introduction to the HBD Reset   13

Meet the Authors: Petronella & Lizzie   17

Overview of the Four Phases of HBD   21

HBD in a Nutshell   22

Transformative Results for Everyone   24

Food: Friend & Foe   27

The HBD Lowdown   29

What to Expect   40

HBD Reset Heroes   42

Lizzie's HBD Pantry, Fridge and Freezer Staples   50

Condiments & Stock Recipes   55

PHASE 1 *THE RESET RULES*	**65**
Introduction	66
Soups & Main Meals	77
PHASE 2 *WE'RE READY TO ROLL!*	**93**
Introduction	94
Breakfasts	109
Main Meals	131
The Classics	132
Crowd Pleasers	148
Comfort	164
Simple, Speedy Suppers	180
Good To Go	196
Day 17: The Results of Your Reset	210
Community: The HBD Club	**211**
Acknowledgements & Notes	**212**
Index	**213**

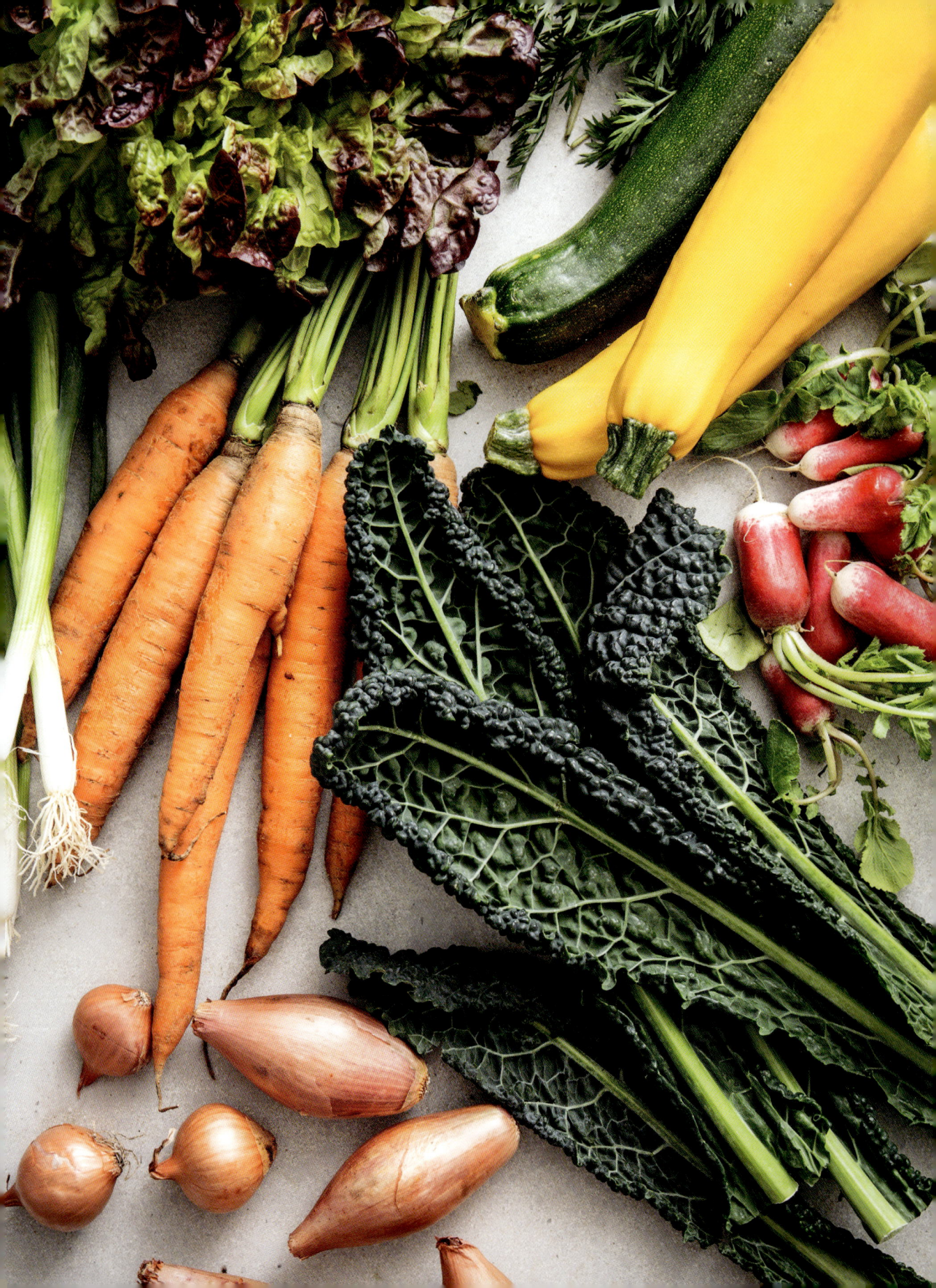

INTRODUCTION

HBD: The Human Being Diet – you'll bless the day you started

HBD, The Human Being Diet, is the joyful and effective antidote to unhealthy fad diets and weight loss jabs, as attested by thousands of happy HBD fans and followers. It describes and explains a simple way of eating for every adult human being (hence the title) who wants to maximise their health and vitality, whether their aim is weight loss or not.

HBD is the healthy and life affirming alternative to GLP-1 weight loss jabs. Originally designed to treat type 2 diabetes, these drugs are the weight loss darlings of the day, but some doctors are urging caution. In February 2025 the BMJ reported 82 deaths related to GLP-1 drugs.[1] Not just 'adverse side effects' – which can include, among others, nausea, vomiting, pancreatitis, intestinal inflammation, dehydration and delirium, as well as constipation, diarrhoea and pain (including heartburn) and gallbladder dysfunction – but *deaths*.[2,3]

Miracle slimming drugs certainly have a record of unpleasant side effects. About 70 percent of GLP-1 users are said to discontinue the drugs after two years because they find the nausea and/or diarrhoea unbearable.[4]

The GLP-1 hormone, which is naturally produced in our intestines when we eat, is only in circulation naturally for about two minutes. When GLP-1 is released, it improves insulin sensitivity, reduces appetite and makes us feel 'full' – all good and beneficial effects for weight loss and overall health. The effect of GLP-1 drugs however, is to keep this hormone in circulation for seven days, rather than two minutes, hence the weekly injections. The long-term health effects of artificially and drastically increasing GLP-1 are unknown. We are playing with fire.

The great news is that we can naturally increase our GLP-1 levels by changing what we eat and without resorting to these drugs and their potentially horrible side effects. We can increase GLP-1 by restricting starchy carbs, by improving our microbiome/gut health, by eating good-quality protein, by getting more fibre and eating more fermented foods, including sauerkraut, kimchi and tempeh. In other words, we can increase it by eating the HBD way and you'll discover another magical hack to improve your GLP-1 levels within this book – spoiler alert... it's apple cider vinegar!

> *Karen: 'I started your HBD plan on 2nd Feb weighing 11 stone 1lb (70kg). Today I'm at 8 stone 9lb (55kg) and have reversed my diabetes. Thank you, I have fully embraced my new lifestyle change and I love your recipes.'*

If weight loss – or the beginnings of type 2 diabetes – is what's attracted you to HBD, the fact you've got this book in your hands means that you've either ruled out using GLP-1 medications as undesirable drugs with unknown long-term side effects, or you've already tried them and realised they're not for you. The problem with magic bullet tactics, aside from the potential side effects and health risks, is that they don't change our relationship with food. Neither do weight loss diets. They don't teach us anything about how our diet affects the way we feel, or which foods best suit us as individuals. Sadly and inevitably, once the diet or treatment is stopped, the weight that's been lost may just as quickly reappear.

HBD resets our relationship with food and we learn which foods best suit us personally. One of the sentiments that's most often shared with me, apart from, 'I only wish I'd discovered this years ago' is, 'I never ever want to go back to how I felt pre HBD – I will never go back to eating like I used to.' And you won't either. You will look back and bless the day you started HBD.

WEIGHT LOSS IS A SIDE EFFECT OF IMPROVED HEALTH

Weight loss is just one of the benefits of adopting HBD and changing the way we eat. In fact weight loss with HBD occurs as a *side effect* of reduced inflammation, rebalanced hormones and blood sugar and improved gut health. We can choose to be lean, with vibrantly good energy and great health. Or thin with a grey pallor, less muscle mass and fragile bones. But be prepared for friends to suspect you of succumbing to the jabs once you start to change before their eyes, despite your newly found HBD glow!

When we follow HBD, and combine good-quality protein with vegetables in three daily meals, and when we fast for at least five hours between meals, our blood sugar stabilises. Stable blood sugar results in diminished hunger and fewer cravings, a sunnier mood, deeper sleep and better energy. We feel liberated! Chronic inflammation – which afflicts many of us – naturally subsides. Chronic inflammation is recognised as the culprit in all the so-called lifestyle diseases, from type 2 diabetes to autoimmune disorders. As well as reduced inflammation, hormones including insulin are brought back into balance, and a side effect of all these benefits is achieving and maintaining a healthy weight.

HBD is a tried and tested approach with thousands of happy fans and followers who have not only achieved their ideal weight and improved their health, but who are also getting more joy out of life. It comprises four phases and ten golden rules and for success with the programme, my first book, *The Human Being Diet* is required reading – it's your indispensable guide to long-term success with HBD. This book, the *HBD Reset Cookbook*, is a treasure trove of recipes, foodie inspiration, cooking techniques and tips, and is designed to help you navigate the trickiest part of the programme, the 16 day Reset. It's your friendly guide and companion and shows you how the HBD lifestyle can be fully integrated into day-to-day life. Prepare to be blown away and delighted by Lizzie's recipes!

> **Suzy:** '*I had my annual bloods taken for my chronic illnesses and I wanted to share with you that I am no longer pre-diabetic and my cholesterol has come down significantly and I'm now in the normal range since starting HBD.*'

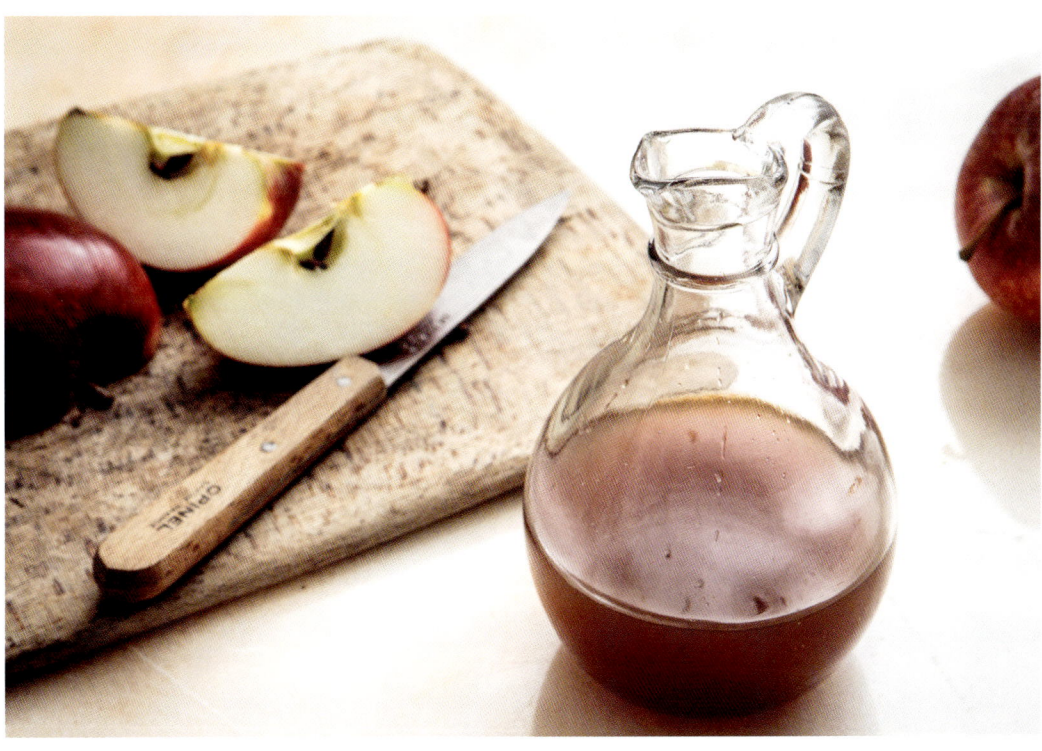

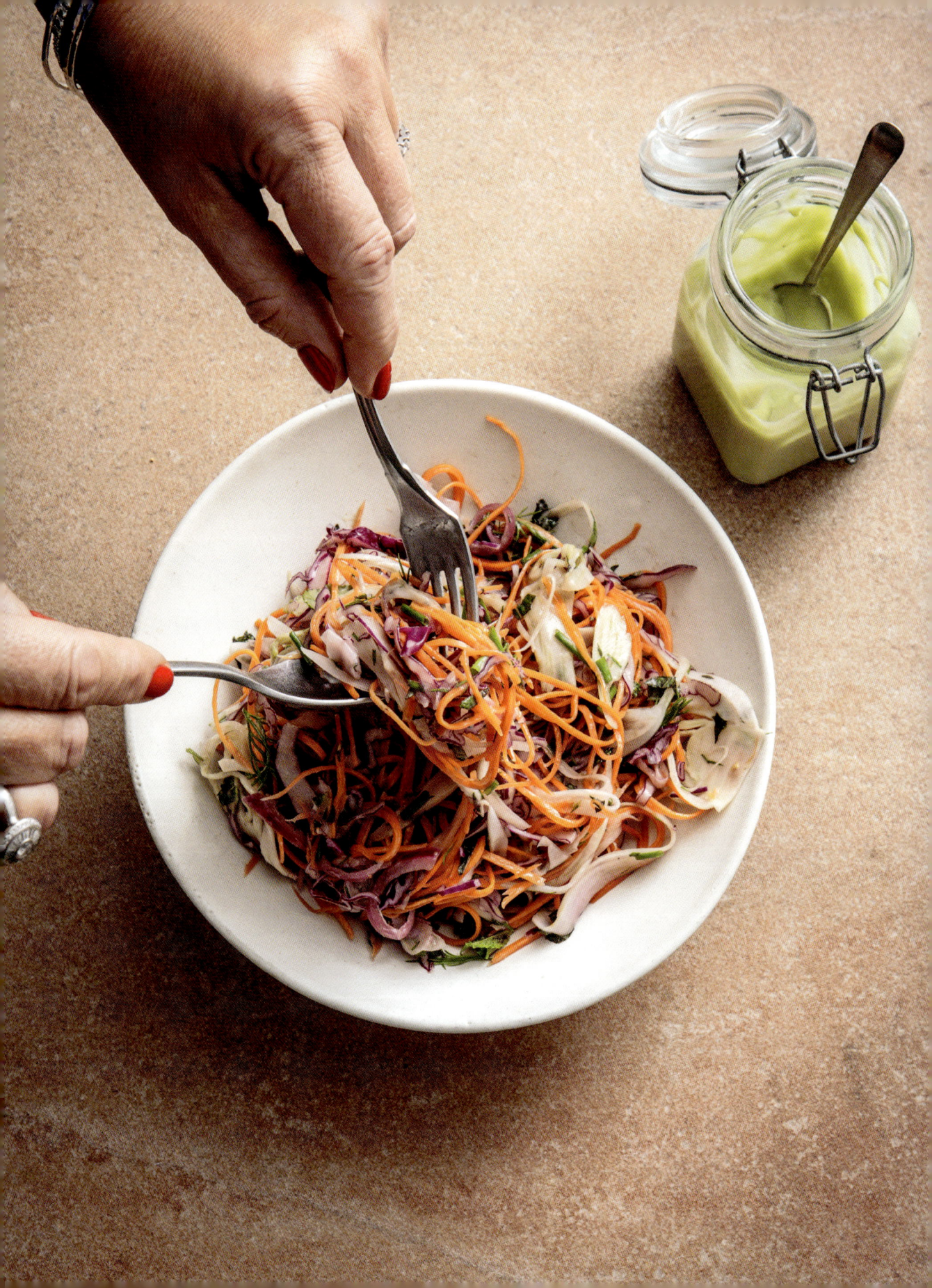

Introduction to the HBD Reset

Chances are you've already discovered The Human Being Diet (HBD) and that you've fallen on this book with a whoop of joy! You already know about the miraculous effects of HBD – from the famous HBD glow, to the boundless energy and deeply refreshing sleep, to the incomparable feeling of lightness and vitality that it delivers. You may have already completed the Reset a few times but *this* time you're planning your Reset happy in the knowledge that, thanks to Lizzie's easy and delectable recipes, it's set to be a delicious one. It's going to be a *feast*!

Every year, each time you recalibrate and reset with HBD, you'll have this indispensable companion by your side. This marks the end to beige/greige food and welcomes in an explosion of taste and colour. Because every day should be a delicious day of wholesome, nutrient-packed food to make you feel as good on the inside as you look on the outside.

If you're new to HBD a brief outline of the four phases and ten rules is included here. To really 'get' the programme and to understand the rules and rationale that set you up for super-success, my first book, *The Human Being Diet*, as mentioned before, is required reading. Read it once and as soon as you've finished, read it again! While you're reading that book you're communicating with your subconscious – you're laying the groundwork, you're explaining to yourself what is to come and you are cementing your commitment to the programme, as well as to yourself. You're going to be giving this your all.

There's nothing to stop you using the 16 day Reset to help you lose weight and feel fabulous for a big birthday or any other festive event. But that's not why I wrote *The Human Being Diet* – the clue is in the title. 'Diet' in its original sense means 'way of life' or lifestyle – as in the Mediterranean diet. HBD is not a quick fix or an unsustainable way of eating that's followed for a limited time with the sole aim of weight loss. As Lizzie says in her introduction (see page 18), HBD describes a new way of eating and living that lasts forever.

What does 'The Human Being' part of the title mean? It means that this way of eating – this way of life – is suitable for every adult human being. We learn, by reading the books and by tuning in to feedback from our bodies, how to eat to feel and look as good as we possibly can. Lizzie's recipes demonstrate that eating well the HBD way is a joyful affair; there's nothing boring or difficult about it. HBD is for every human being who wants to get the most joy out of life and every human being who cares about their current and future health.

Phases 1 and 2 are collectively known as the Reset. The 16 days of the Reset are the most challenging, but also the most important and most rewarding part of HBD – they lay the solid foundation and set the scene for long term, enduring success. Every day of the Reset must be treated as sacrosanct, and the 16 days need to be completed without interruption. Falling off the wagon or cheating means starting all over again. The first 16 days are tough, the rules are rigid – and this period is vitally important because it acts to reset our metabolism. It's during the Reset that we make the switch to burning fat instead of sugar and carbs for energy: we remind out bodies how to do it.

That's why Lizzie and I wrote this book – it's all about supporting you through the Reset. We want to set you up for huge success, so you are ready and excited to continue with the rest of the programme, having experienced the most delicious first 16 days and feeling so much better in such a short time. Our aim is to get this most challenging and most important part of your HBD adventure off to a thrilling start – to make it as simple and easy for you as we possibly can.

The Reset is followed by ten weeks of Phase 3, Burn (those with more weight to lose continue in Burn until they reach their goal). Burn is a continuation of what you've been doing in the Reset with the glorious addition of extra virgin olive oil and a weekly treat meal – and there's chocolate too! So 12 weeks in total before you head into Phase 4, the forever phase, because experts agree that it generally takes about three months to establish and embed new habits.

For even more support treat yourself to a copy of *The HBD Cookbook*, which contains fabulous recipes for all four phases and consider joining us in The HBD Club – for community, live clinics and Q&A. It's a really inspiring and friendly place to be and it's also where we hold guided Resets, which take place in January, March or April (depending on Easter) and September each year.

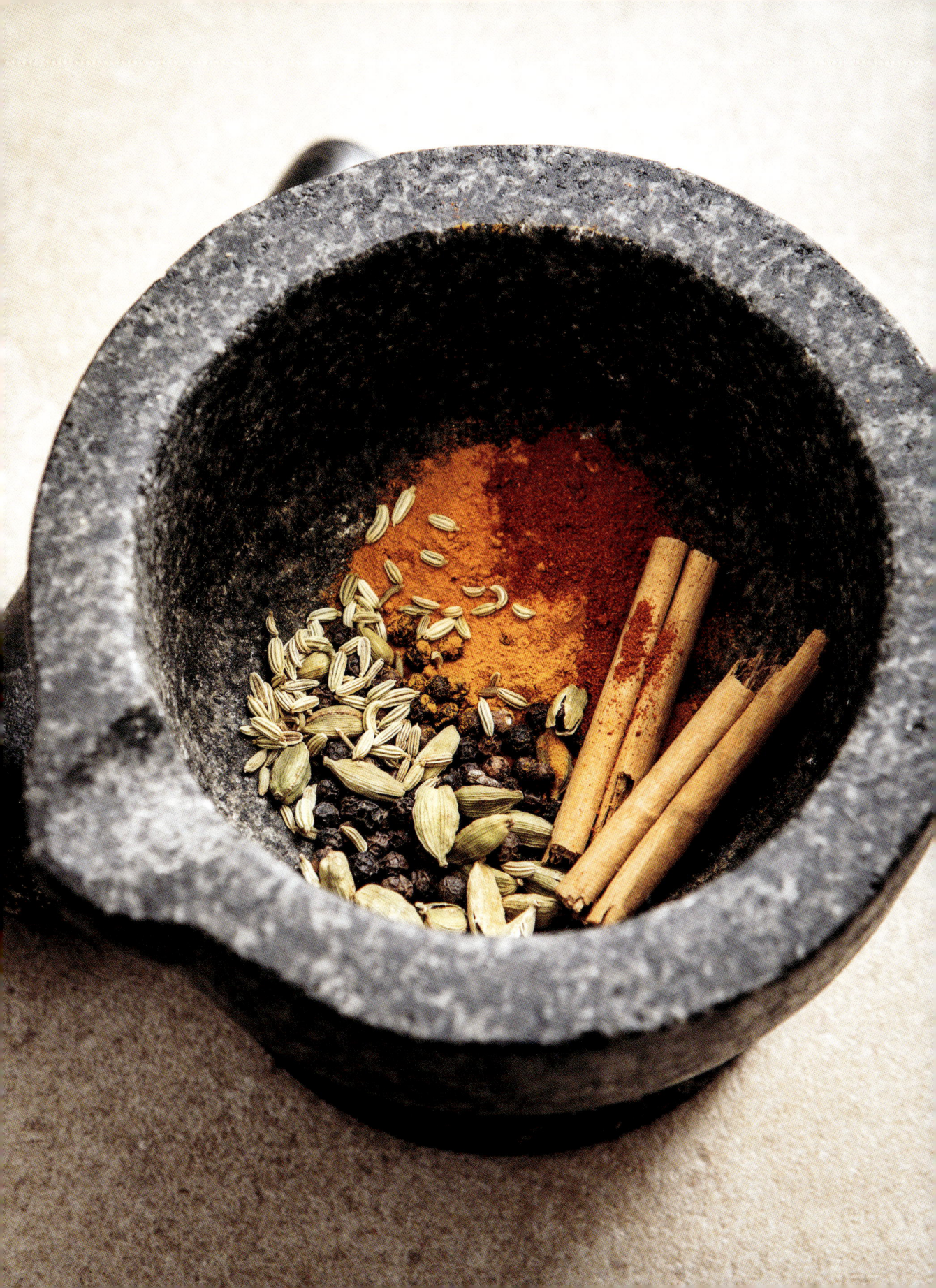

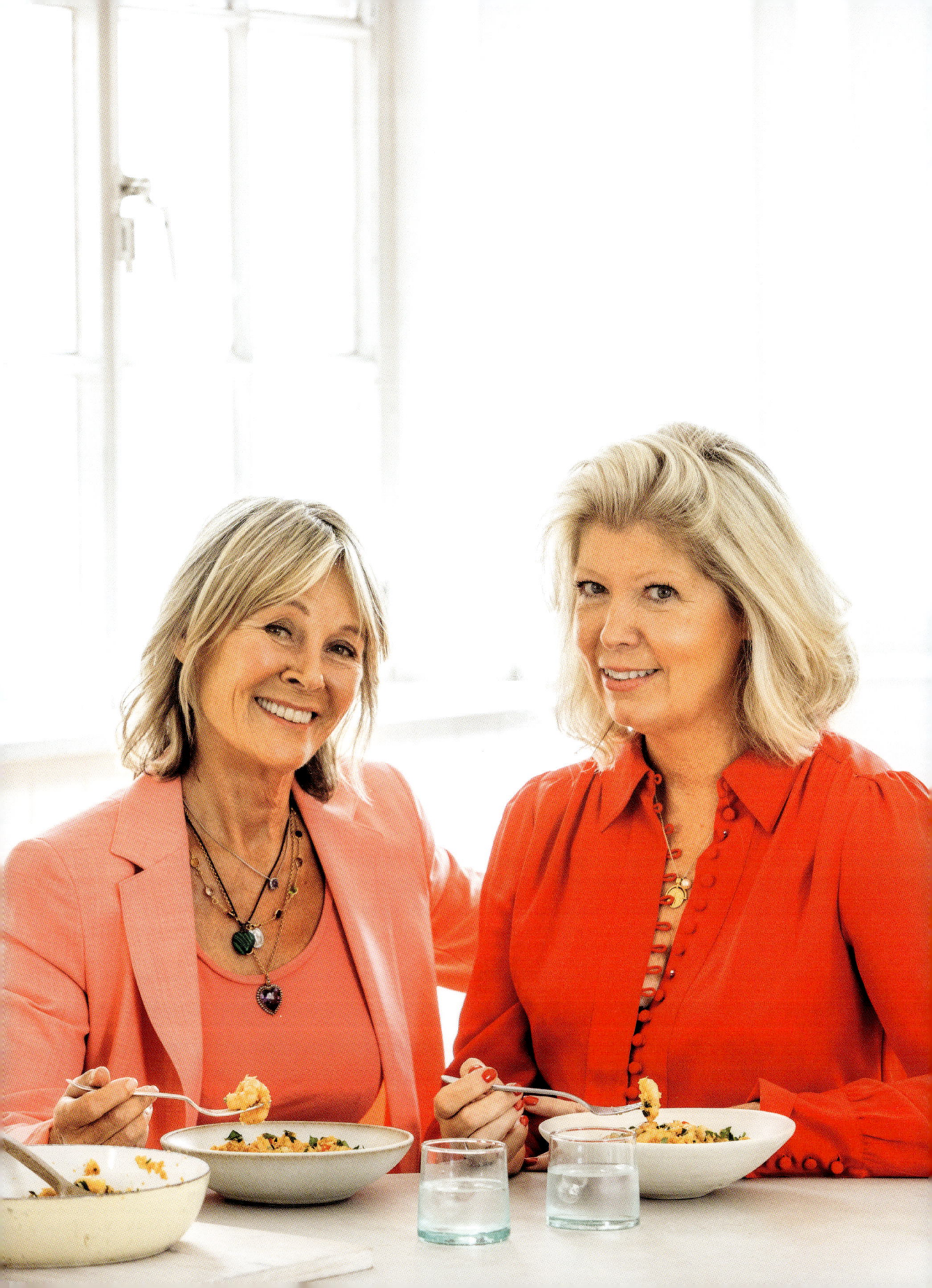

Meet the Authors: Petronella & Lizzie

PETRONELLA

I first started being fascinated with nutrition when my son had been prescribed countless courses of antibiotics for respiratory tract infections. The antibiotics were only making things worse – he was ill more and more often. It wasn't until we took him off wheat and dairy and introduced probiotics that he began to recover. It was as if someone had turned the lights on and I could see the direction my life would take. I enrolled in London's Institute for Optimal Nutrition (ION).

Ah-ha moments in nutrition

Following three years of fascinating lectures, case studies and practical experiments, and after graduating from ION, I opened my own practice in Chelsea, where I worked for twenty years. I gained a stellar reputation (and a long waiting list) for helping people overcome chronic skin, digestive and weight problems, and became known as one of London's top nutritionists.

Writing the book

It was the waiting list, in a roundabout way, that prompted me to write my first book, *The Human Being Diet*. What do you do when there aren't enough hours in the day to see the people who want to come to your clinic? And what about the people who wanted to know how to feel better but couldn't afford to see a nutritionist?

I realised the answer was to write a book. I started work distilling everything I'd learned, from years of invaluable clinical experience, numerous courses, reading and doing my own research, into my first book, *The Human Being Diet*.

I aimed to write a book that could be used by anyone who cared about their health and wanted to maximise their energy, solve their niggling health problems and get more joy out of life, whether they wanted to lose weight or not. The book contained an easy to follow framework with clear and simple guidelines for success.

Lizzie & The HBD Club

The reason this is called the Human Being Diet is because it's for every adult – man or woman – who wants to feel better and get more joy out of life; it's not just for women.

Earlier in 2025 we created The HBD Club, which is a membership club hosted on the specialist community platform Circle. We hold weekly live clinics and Q&A sessions, and we have a fabulous collection of resources, including an ever expanding recipe collection, thanks to our HBD Angel, Elisabeth Whiting (Lizzie).

Lizzie's recipes have been going down a storm in the club – she is a talented foodie and her recipes are easy to follow and absolutely delicious. As an added bonus, she's a joyously uplifting friend. I was thrilled to be asked by Katya Shipster at HarperCollins to write a new cookbook – and doubly thrilled when Lizzie agreed to co-author it and create the recipes.

You might think, with not one but two cookbooks to my name, that I'm a bit of a foodie. I'm really not, although I do love good food and eating out.

During our annual HBD Reset it's generally me cooking in the kitchen. Until our Reset this year it was a pretty joyless affair. My husband Riccardo is always kind about what I'm serving, despite the dreariness of it. Happily all that changed this year when we guzzled our way through Lizzie's delicious recipes for our Reset – the food was much more interesting!

Lizzie has been a passionate and creative cook all her life. She is fascinated by taking simple, fresh ingredients and turning them into something magical; she has relished the challenge of creating delicious HBD recipes. Happily for us, this Reset cookbook was her genius idea, as you'll find out below!

> **Debbie Roper featured in the** *Telegraph* **when she lost more than 2 stone (12.7kg) and went from a size 14 to a size 8:** **'I'm thrilled to report the eating plan has changed my whole life. The menopause doesn't mean weight gain is inevitable. Just as I was inspired to change my life by reading about someone (Cath Weller) in this paper, I'd love it if someone else who was perhaps feeling "invisible" in the menopause, might see they can change their body and their outlook just like I have'.**

LIZZIE'S STORY – HEDONIST TO HEALTHY
A FOODIE'S TALE OF JOY AND FEASTING OVER FAMINE

I *really* love food. I feel absolute joy, deep in my soul as I loiter at the fish counter. The consequence of being so in love with food is that just after my fiftieth birthday I realised I had become rather rotund. One of my biggest joys in life – food – had become the enemy. I was also often tired, my joints ached and my brain fog was off the charts.

A wake-up call

I then had a huge wake-up call when my glamorous and wonderful mum died suddenly. She too was a true *bon vivant* – but this led to health problems and a tragically untimely death at 74. I didn't want my children to go through such a monumental loss too soon. It was time to take control of my eating and health.

With so many diet plans out there, I was uncertain where to start: I needed a new way of eating that was sustainable, healthy and most importantly, delicious and satisfying. I wanted desperately to be allowed a social life – to have precious time feasting on my favourite foods with my fabulous, feisty and fascinating girlfriends.

Discovering HBD

In autumn 2022, I bumped into a great friend and did a double take; she had always been gorgeous, but now she looked incredible. She was glowing, super slim and looked ten years younger. She confided that she had lost more than 2.5 stone (16kg) in a few months, but most startling was how healthy she looked. Her skin was amazing, hair glossy and eyes bright. Her secret was Petronella's HBD.

So in January 2023 I started my first reset with huge trepidation. I was terrified of being hungry and even more worried about failing. However, by day two of Phase 2 (P2) my mindset began to change. This was do-able, the key was to take it one day at a time and to remember that it was only for 16 days. Already my clothes felt less tight.

During that first Reset I lost a staggering 6kg in 16 days. My brain fog lifted, my bones stopped aching and I was sleeping better than I had in decades. My taste buds were recharged and simple food tasted amazing – my fridge-cold apple was a taste sensation. This was not the terrifying journey of deprivation I had so feared; I was loving food in an entirely new way.

Reset complete, I was hooked. I felt re-energised, and already had the famous HBD glow: bring on Phase 3. But how could I ensure that HBD would be sustainable longer term? Living in a busy house full of hungry teenagers and animals, I needed to create family favourites that we could all eat together – meals that were quick to prepare and 100 percent HBD friendly, albeit with extra carbs on the side for them.

We were all raising our nutritional game together. My children loved the greater variety and more interesting food in their diet. It gave me a sense of joy, and serving truly nourishing food to my loved ones was an act of love in itself. I developed different ways to cook food to accommodate the HBD way of life and ensure delicious textures and flavours.

My repertoire of recipes grew and in spring 2023 Petronella invited me to join her on Instagram. I was honoured and a little star struck; however, she was so warm and supportive that I thoroughly enjoyed myself. We stayed in touch and Petronella asked if I would be interested in contributing to her fantastic new HBD Club that launched in January 2025 and then to this cookbook too.

> *I am excited about the future. There will undoubtedly be rosé and breadbaskets in my future; life is short! But now they are reserved for treat meals and holidays. The physical and emotional balance that an HBD lifestyle provides is priceless. I feel stronger, my energy levels are better, my aches have gone and I sleep soundly.*
>
> *For me, HBD has become our family norm. It no longer feels challenging or scary and there is no going back.*

MIDLIFE MAYHEM

Lizzie's story may strike a chord with many of us – showing how food, which was always such a pleasure, can become the enemy. Also showing how at midlife our bodies change, our microbiome changes, our metabolism seems to slow down and we can no longer eat in the way we always have. The treachery of it! As many of us have ruefully discovered, me included, counting and cutting calories doesn't help and neither do torturous gym sessions or long runs. How about the advice to eat less and exercise more if you want to lose weight? It doesn't work, not in midlife anyway, and an inability to lose weight can make us feel frauds and failures.

We need to improve our gut health and that of our microbiome, reduce inflammation and get our insulin and blood sugar levels under control. We're definitely not counting calories (or macros) with HBD but we are making every calorie count. We're getting rid of sugars and refined carbs – all those empty calories – which rob us of energy and nutrients, and we're choosing to return to health. We're eating three meals a day and fasting for at least five hours between each meal.

Meal by delicious meal and day by day we're looking after our health. As Lizzie has written in her introduction, we're also looking after ourselves for the people we most love – we want to be around for them, and feeling as well as we possibly can, for as long as we can. It's so simple when we know how. Let's avoid the emulsifiers, the additives and preservatives and fake flavours of ultra-processed foods (UPF) and celebrate nature's bounty and our revitalised taste buds – yes, prepare to be amazed by how alive you will feel and how exciting your food will taste just a few days in!

But this doesn't mean you can't have any fun and go wild with food sometimes. HBD feasting (the weekly treat meal from Phase 3 onwards) is one of the rules and a vital part of the programme. The weekly glut of extra food – mainly in the form of fats – serves three purposes:

- We snap the body out of fasting/detox mode, which encourages it to burn more fat.
- A little poison, aka hormesis, is revitalising and perks up the immune system.
- Pleasure is good for us! Tribal feasting with our friends and relatives is deep in our DNA.

Overview of the Four Phases of HBD

Phase 1:
Two days of vegetables only. No pulses, no protein, no grains, no alcohol, no sugars or sweeteners, no dairy and no fruit.

Phase 2:
Fourteen days of eating three meals a day with a five hour fast (water only) between each meal. Phase 2 is grain, alcohol, oil, sugar and sweetener free. You can introduce fruit in Phase 2 but the only compulsory fruit is your daily apple. It's not a rule but it's recommended that you avoid dairy (cheese, yoghurt) before reintroducing it in Phase 3. Milk is off the menu for everyone. You are also recommended, particularly if anything hurts, or if you have any digestive problems, to avoid nightshades (more about dairy and nightshades in Potentially Problematic Foods below).

We've included some information on Phase 3 and Phase 4 so you have an idea of what's to come, but the information below doesn't apply to the Reset.

Phase 3 Burn:
Ten weeks minimum. This is an extension of Phase 2 – three meals a day with five hour fasts between – but with the joyful addition of extra virgin olive oil and a weekly treat meal. Phase 3 also includes optional rye bread and dark chocolate. This is when dairy and nightshades can be reintroduced and reactions monitored. Additional foods, including more starchy vegetables, can now also be added.

Phase 4:
The forever phase. With valuable lessons learnt thanks to feedback from your body in Phase 3, HBD becomes your new way of living and your forever lifestyle.

HBD in a Nutshell

So what is HBD – what's it all about? If a friend were to ask you to sum it up, you might explain it like this:

It's a take on the Mediterranean diet – the focus is on wholesome wholefoods. The first 16 days (aka The Reset) are very strict: oil, alcohol, sugar (including honey and sweeteners) and grains are all off limits. It involves eating three meals a day with a fast of at least five hours between each meal. Tea and coffee can be drunk, black and unsweetened, with meals only. Between meals you just drink lots and lots of water (still or sparkling).

One type of good-quality protein (e.g. eggs, meat, fish, chicken or tofu) and a mixture of at least three different types of vegetables are included in each meal and everything is weighed before it's cooked. The only compulsory fruit, from day 3 onwards, is one apple a day. HBD can be followed by omnivores, vegetarians and vegans – every adult human who cares about their health, whether they want to lose weight or not. It's the antithesis of a fad diet. There are no meal replacements, bars or shakes, no calorie (or macro) counting and no gimmicks – it's a simple and wholesome way of eating.

> **Cath Weller in the** *Telegraph*: 'The other bonus has been the way my energy has sky-rocketed. Matt, my husband, will say: "Gosh Cath, where are you getting it from?" Eating well and staying away from processed food has definitely helped. I feel renewed. I'd battled my relationship with food for so many years and now I'm healthy and I feel fantastic. It's a feeling that money can't buy.'

One more thing that's off limits during the Reset is intense or cardio exercise. Petronella explains in her book *The Human Being Diet* that this kind of exercise acts as a stressor and pushes us into the sympathetic nervous system (aka fight or flight) and increases the stress hormone cortisol.

She says to view the reset as a period of readjustment – a time to bring everything back into balance.

The Reset is the toughest part of the programme, but by day 16 you'll feel lighter and brighter than you have in years – and that inspires you and motivates you to keep going. Successfully completing the Reset gives you such a feeling of pride and such a sense of achievement. Everything's easier after the first 16 days of the Reset and by the end of it you'll already have the beginnings of the HBD glow – and you'll feel so much better.

In Phase 3, which lasts for at least ten weeks – longer if you've got more weight to lose – you have extra virgin olive oil (a tablespoon with every meal) for its incredible health-giving properties. Extra virgin olive oil is the star of the Mediterranean diet and has amazingly powerful fat-burning and heart-health effects. You can also have a couple of squares of 85 percent dark chocolate once a day, and some wholegrain rye bread. But best of all you have a treat meal once a week, when anything goes – this is the feasting part! Lashings of butter and mayo, steak and chips, chocolate mousse and double cream – whatever you like.

Phase 3 segues into Phase 4, the forever phase, when HBD has truly become your new way of life and there's no going back. It's when you realise that eating the HBD way is a no brainer – and you have experienced such profound changes to your energy, your sleep, your feeling of lightness and wellbeing. A return to the old ways of eating and feeling just isn't an option – it's unthinkable! You will forever bless the day that you discovered HBD and, like me, you will want the whole world to know about it because it's so simple and it delivers life changing results!

NON-SCALE VICTORIES

Us HBDers enjoy our non-scale victories (NSVs) as much as we love the weight loss. NSVs include things like deeper sleep, better energy, clearer thinking, glowing skin, less bloating and better digestion, as well as diminished cravings and the incomparable feeling of calm. It's the NSVs that make HBD a non-negotiable, forever lifestyle.

Transformative Results for Everyone

That's no exaggeration: HBD does indeed deliver life-changing results, and we get a steady stream of heartfelt thanks and testimonials from self-proclaimed, proud and happy HBD evangelists! We hear from HBD followers in all phases of the programme about transformative weight loss – it's not unusual for people to lose 6kg (depending on how much they'd like to lose) in the first 16 days of the Reset. We also hear about rebalanced hormones and improvements to skin, energy, mood and sleep, resolution of joint pain and migraines, and even the disappearance of autoimmune antibodies.

Many people come to HBD because they've witnessed the transformation of friends – seen the weight loss, the energy, the HBD glow – and listened to them evangelising about it. But increasingly people are turning to HBD to solve other problems – problems such as aching joints, low mood, lack of energy and unrefreshing sleep.

We hear from people whose blood pressure and cholesterol have normalised and from those whose doctors have reduced or discontinued medication for conditions such as acid reflux and type 2 diabetes. We also receive moving accounts from people who tell us that they feel liberated – people who've suffered from lifelong disordered eating and cycles of bingeing and starving. For the first time in their life they now feel sane about the way they eat; they can enjoy eating once more. The 'food noise' that's plagued them for most of their lives has been silenced at last.

> **Marie: 'From the minute I read your book, I knew the structure and logic would work for me. I had really high blood pressure which the doctors had struggled for years to manage. I had tried every diet known to man and went to the gym regularly but couldn't shift a pound. I started at 10 stone 10lb (68kg) 10 weeks ago with no target until I read the exchange between @mrsaddtobasket and yourself about not limiting yourself. Today I weighed in at 8 stone 13lb (56.6kg) just 10 weeks later and my blood pressure is the lowest it's ever been and my medication is currently being reviewed.**

That one approach can have such wide-ranging beneficial effects is evidence of the curative power of real food. We can base our diet on ultra-processed factory food (UPF) to keep us alive, or we can choose to thrive by feeding our bodies, our microbiome and our brain food that is minimally processed, nutrient-dense and wholesome. This Hippocrates saying may be thousands of years old, but it's as true today as it ever was: 'Let food be your medicine and medicine be your food'. Our good health, current and future, is in our hands and we can absolutely choose what's on our plate and how we feed ourselves.

> **Melanie:** *'This lifestyle, not a diet, has changed my life. As with many others who have come across HBD, shared by its creator the lovely Petronella, I discovered it in 2022 after seeing Instagram posts from @mrsaddtobasket (Cath Weller). I have battled an eating disorder since the age of 15 – years of starving and over-exercising that unhealthily "worked" during my 20s, 30s, but when I reached my 40s it just wasn't working any more. I was not in a happy place with myself or my relationship with food. I took the plunge (I did not do the salts as I didn't want to awaken past laxative abuse). The weight fell off and due to my past history, I was getting a few concerned comments from family and friends. My husband was my biggest backup and reassured everyone that he had never seen me eat so much and so regularly in 25 years. My energy levels were through the roof, along with great mood, the aches and pains from the menopause disappeared, and I got that famous HBD glow. Roll on to today and I have just completed my first Reset and yes I did the salts for myself – that is a huge achievement mentally. My mind, and my relationship with food, has completely changed; food is medicine and not the devil.'*

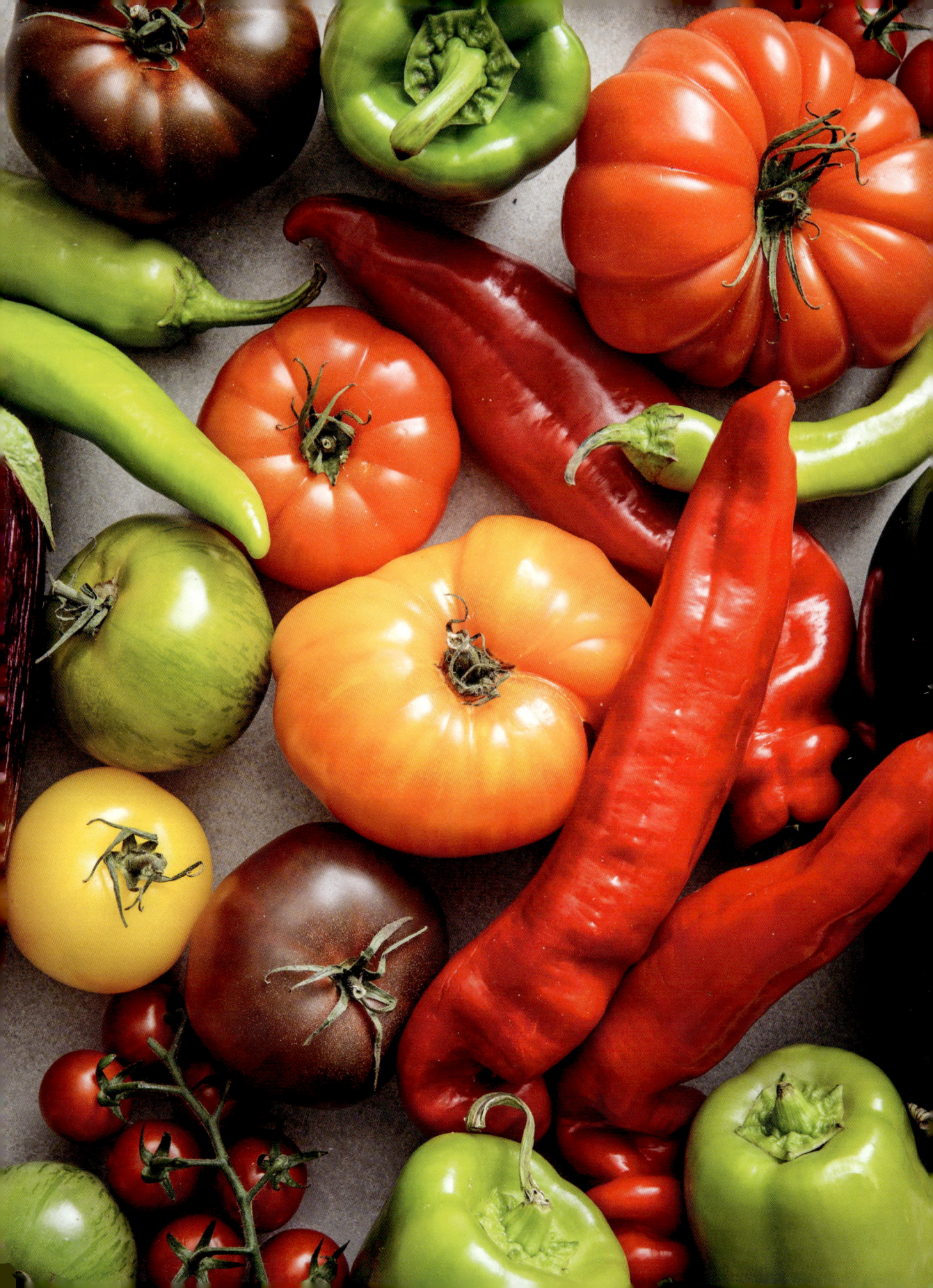

Food: Friend & Foe

Food is not just fuel, and it's more than the protein, fat, carbs and calories it delivers. It carries information into our cells – it speaks to our DNA. Our food has the potential to silence the genes associated with inflammation and all our modern lifestyle diseases – or to activate them. What we eat doesn't change the sequence of our genes – our DNA – but it does have a crucial effect, in a process known as epigenetics, on affecting how our genes are expressed (when they are turned on and off). The right food – real food – gives our bodies and brains what they need for optimal function.

The alarming rise in our reliance on convenient ultra-processed, factory-made food for sustenance is rightly blamed for fuelling the explosion of inflammatory diseases, long term chronic health conditions and obesity that is blighting so many lives. It's time to return to eating the foods that made us human, the food that speaks to our genes and which delivers the nutrients we need for health and happiness.

Food can act both as a medicine and as a poison. Food can be defined as: a nutritious substance that provides living organisms with energy and which sustains processes, including growth and repair, that are essential to life. So food sustains life. The definition of poison is: a destructive or harmful substance that through its chemical action kills, injures or impairs living organisms – poison destroys life.

I and many HBDers have discovered that wheat acts more like a poison than a food in our bodies. Others make similar discoveries when it comes to certain nightshade vegetables or to dairy foods; one man's meat really is another man's poison.

During the course of HBD and especially when you move from Phase 2 to Phase 3 and reintroduce certain foods, you'll discover which ones suit you personally and which are best left alone. Some of us do just fine on dairy and grains, and on nightshades such as tomatoes and peppers (see Potentially Problematic Foods, page 32). But sometimes the feedback from your body when you reintroduce certain foods can be alarming

> ***Annie: 'After following HBD for 9 months I am no longer pre diabetic (HbA1c is now 38 down from 42) and my cholesterol is down massively too. I really can't thank you enough and, give or take the odd kilo, I've maintained my weight through Phase 4 despite holidays and celebrations! I feel so motivated and my way of thinking about food has totally shifted. I thought I had a healthy diet but now I know my portions were too large and I snacked.'***

Dr Jenni Byrom: 'Petronella's years of clinical experience and sound scientific research are combined in an effective, easy to follow, no nonsense plan which has enabled my patients to lose necessary weight before surgery and to improve their overall health – highly recommended.'

– you get very clear messages about what it does and doesn't like! Even seemingly innocuous foods, such as sweet potatoes, which we may have been eating regularly for years can turn out to be toxic for us personally. Our brains and bodies really are the best teachers once we learn to tune in and listen to the messages.

Despite the title of his book *Food Isn't Medicine* and his advice to 'give ourselves permission to eat all foods' Dr Joshua Wolrich shed four stone (25.4kg) by changing his diet. He swapped sandwiches, crisps, chocolates, pasta and greasy fry-ups for nutritious home cooked meals. He wanted to be a better example to his patients. When interviewed by the *Daily Mail* three years before his book came out, he said: 'it's all about focusing on balanced, nutrient dense foods and addressing disordered eating behaviour – rather than on filling up on food that doesn't do anything for your health.' Food really *is* medicine!

The HBD Lowdown

IS HBD A LOW CARB REGIME?

Let's dig into the nitty gritty! We need protein and fat for life itself – we can't survive without these two macronutrients. Do we need carbs to sustain life? No! Do we need carbs to keep us healthy? Absolutely! But not the refined, fibreless carbs in sugar and white flour. What we need is the carbs with benefits – the vegetables and a little fruit that come wrapped up with fibre, vitamins and minerals, along with plant antioxidants, the polyphenols.

'Eat the rainbow' is good advice – the beautiful plant pigments, all the different colours, bring unique health benefits. Just like plants, we need water, food and sun to flourish and thrive. Plants get their food from the soil – their roots take up and incorporate minerals such as calcium, iron and magnesium into the plants themselves. We, in turn get the nutrients we need by eating plants and by eating the animals that feed on the plants.

All carbohydrates, apart from fibre, ultimately break down to sugar – it's essentially the speed with which the body turns them into sugar that makes them good or bad for us. HBD is not a low carb regime, but it is low in simple and starchy carbs. You've probably heard that we have to eat carbs for energy – that's just not true – but what we do need them for (the right kind of course) is the health of our gut and our microbes. And when we have a healthy gut and happy, perky microbes we are happy and healthy too!

A quick guide to carbs

- **Sugars:** simple carbs/natural sugars found in fruit juice and soft drinks, and added sugars including sugar itself (honey, syrups and nectars).

- **Starches:** refined and complex carbs, found in pulses (peas, beans and lentils), grains, fruit, corn, root veg and potatoes – starches are long chains of sugar molecules.

- **Fibre:** found in complex carbs such as pulses, vegetables, wholegrains, nuts and seeds, and fruit. Fibre itself doesn't break down to sugar because we can't digest it, but fibre is food for our microbes.

Simple sugars, as well as potatoes, refined and starchy grains, and excessive fruit, are the carbs associated with inflammation and creeping weight gain. Sugar and refined carbs are 'anti-nutrients'. They burn through our valuable vitamins and minerals, including B vitamins and vitamin C, as well as magnesium and chromium when they're processed in our bodies. They give us nothing in return other than a quick energy burst, which is quickly followed by an energy slump. They have an overall negative impact on our mood and our energy and, by increasing insulin and inflammation, make weight loss next to impossible.

Starchy carbs, apart from pulses (beans and lentils), are mostly off the menu in the Reset – we're minimising sugars, including fruit sugars, and encouraging our bodies to burn fat and to reduce inflammation. Once we get to Phase 3 we can experiment by adding starchier carbs again, such as 100 percent rye bread (or buckwheat, for those who can't tolerate rye/gluten) sweet potatoes and other root vegetables.

Fibre-rich complex carbs as found in root veg, pulses and wholegrains, are associated with general good health and a healthy microbiome. Remember that all carbs, other than fibre, break down to sugar and stimulate insulin release. The more fibre a food contains, the longer it takes to digest, and the less impact it has on our blood sugar and insulin levels. And that's a good thing.

PROTEIN

Protein is more complicated. All we really need to know about it is which foods are good protein sources, e.g. fish, meat, poultry, eggs, tofu and tempeh, and that eating enough protein keeps us feeling full for longer. It's particularly important, especially for weight loss, to eat good-quality protein for breakfast. HBD advice is to eat breakfast within an hour of waking.

The protein we eat is digested and broken down into single amino acids, or short chains of them, which are then rearranged by our body into the proteins that we need. All the different proteins that make up our bones, muscles, skin, hair and all our hormones and immune cells, are made from the protein that we eat. So that expression, 'You are what you eat' really is true.

Of the 20 amino acids we need, nine are termed 'essential'. We must get these nine from our diet, and from these we can make all the other necessary proteins. Foods that contain these nine amino acids in the right ratios are called 'complete' or 'high value' proteins. Complete proteins are supplied by eggs, fish, poultry, meat, dairy foods and soy. Soy is the only complete, high value vegan protein. If you're sleuthing on the internet for more information on this, you might see these complete proteins referred to as being of 'high biological value'.

Protein plant foods such as pulses (peas, beans, chickpeas and lentils) as well as nuts and seeds contain 'incomplete proteins'. Although quinoa – not included in HBD, other than at treat meals, until Phase 4 – is often billed as a protein food, it actually contains roughly five times more carbohydrate than protein. It's not a protein, it's a carb with good PR! In its defence, quinoa does contain all the essential amino acids we need, but not in meaningful amounts. Legumes, including beans, chickpeas and lentils, are known as plant proteins, but all, apart from soy, are more carb than protein.

Mixing our proteins, whether mixing complete and incomplete proteins, always results in our body absorbing less protein and creating more waste. So what happens to the aminos we're not able to use? They break down into toxic ammonia and then urea and are finally peed out with the help of our kidneys. Grains and beans are the real culprits when it comes to over acidifying our bodies, because so much of their protein is 'wasted'. You can read more about this, and the 'biological value' of protein, if it interests you, in *The Human Being Diet*.

FATS

The essential fats – 'essential' meaning the ones we must include in our diet – are the omega-3 and 6 families. These fats are supplied by eggs, fish and meat as well as by nuts and seeds. They are vital for our health, for our brain and eyes, and for our immune system and hormones – and they help to regulate inflammation.

We are not good at converting the omega-3 in plant foods such as flaxseeds and walnuts into the highly anti-inflammatory long chain EPA and DHA fats that are vitally important for our health. These fats are naturally found in fish, shellfish and algae, and to a lesser extent in grass-fed dairy and meat. In fact, it's impossible to get the necessary EPA and DHA from vegetarian food – we can only get these omega-3s from fish, or fish oil or algae supplements. In other words, plant-based folk, and anyone who doesn't eat fish, really must supplement with these oils for their health.

Unlike omega-3, omega-6 has both pro and anti-inflammatory properties. It can be converted into GLA, a potent anti-inflammatory, but only if the enzymes for the conversion are present and working as they should. Anthropologists tell us that until a hundred years ago, the ratio of omega-6 to omega-3 in our diet was less than 4:1 – but in a typical modern diet today, the ratio is 20:1.

'Reducing the omega-6/3 ratio, particularly through reductions in the intake of refined omega-6 seed oil, and increasing the intake of marine omega-3s, either through dietary means or supplementation, may be an effective strategy for reducing inflammation, allergies, and autoimmune reactions.' (Dr James DiNicolantonio 2021) In other words, once we get rid of the high omega-6 vegetable and seed oils (e.g. rapeseed and sunflower oil) and eat more oily fish (salmon, sardines, mackerel) or supplement with omega-3, our health improves.

POTENTIALLY PROBLEMATIC FOODS

We're not talking about ultra-refined factory made foods, or the ubiquitous vegetable/seed oils, or sugar, or wheat or refined carbs here, all of which are off the menu for the Reset. This is about two food groups, dairy and nightshades, which many of us may regularly include in our diet, but which just might be sapping our energy, adding to inflammation and preventing us from feeling as well as we possibly can.

Dairy

If you've already completed a dairy-free HBD Reset, and you reintroduced it in Phase 3 and know you're OK with it, feel free to include full-fat yoghurt (or cheese) for breakfast and/or cheese for the occasional main meal in your Reset. But if this is your first time with HBD it's strongly recommended that you avoid dairy and see what, if anything, happens when you reintroduce it in Phase3. Many HBDers have been shocked and surprised by their body's reaction to dairy when they reintroduce it. Blocked sinuses, skin breakouts, joint pain, bloating and constipation or diarrhoea, as well as negative changes in mood and energy, are some of the possible effects.

There are two potential problems with dairy. The first is the sugar (lactose), which some of us just cannot digest – mostly we lose our ability to digest it when we grow our milk teeth. An inability to digest lactose can result in wind, bloating and pain. The second is the dairy protein casein, which is a common allergen. All mammals' milk, except for cows' milk, but including human milk, contains A2 casein. A genetic mutation in European cattle, believed to have occurred about 8,000 years ago, resulted in some of these cows producing predominantly A1 instead of A2 milk casein.

If you have already discovered that you are fine with goat or sheep dairy but not with cow it's likely to be due to the better tolerated and more easily digested A2 casein it contains. A2 casein, as well as being the main protein found in sheep and goat dairy, is also in the milk of Jersey, Guernsey, Charolais and Limousin cows. Other cows, including black and white Friesian cows, and also Ayrshire, British Shorthorn and Holstein cows, produce mainly A1 milk casein.

For this reason, you might test sheep or goat's yoghurt or cheese before trying cow dairy when reintroducing dairy in Phase 3, because of the differences in the casein protein. If you're absolutely certain you don't have a problem with dairy – because you eliminated it in a previous Reset, and found you were fine when you reintroduced it in Phase 3 – you could opt for unsweetened, unflavoured full-fat sheep, cow or goat yoghurt with one type of fruit for breakfast (see the Phase 2 food lists). If you do choose to have yoghurt, make sure that it's at least 5g fat and has at least 9g protein and 4g (or less) carbohydrate per 100g. Avoid all low-fat dairy foods.

Nightshades

This food group includes aubergines, tomatoes, peppers and all the red spices made from them (paprika, chilli, cayenne, crushed red peppers) as well as potatoes. Tobacco and ashwagandha are also part of the nightshade family. Some of us are sensitive to some or all nightshade foods and herbs. If anything hurts (joint pain, migraines) or if you have any gut problems (e.g. bloating, IBS) it's important to avoid all these foods and spices through the reset before reintroducing them in Phase 3 and monitoring any reactions. The advice is as for dairy – if you've never eliminated nightshades in the past, consider avoiding them through your Reset.

> *Rachel: 'Just to say thank you for the plan and sharing your brilliant knowledge – have reached my goal and lost 5 stone (32kg) since following your HBD rules. Feel for first time in life (age 59!) I have a clear plan to move forward and maintain it, so a huge* **thank you** *from me!'*

Tomatoes and other nightshades can be included in the Reset if you know they suit you because you have eliminated them for at least 14 days in the past and didn't react badly on reintroduction. If so you can include tinned or fresh tomatoes, but be mindful of the daily limit of 30g. Concentrated tomato paste or purée can also be used, but sparingly – 5g or less per day. Tomatoes are limited because they contains much less fibre and much more fructose (sugar) than green vegetables.

YOUR FOOD DIARY

Getting into the habit of keeping a daily food diary is the single most helpful tool for helping you to stay on track and to pinpoint potentially troublesome foods when you graduate to Phase 3. See page 49 for more information, or *The HBD Journal*.

Track variety in your diet. Avoid repeating a protein food in the same day – so if you have chicken for lunch don't have it again for dinner.

Vegetables – aim for three different veggies with each meal and eat as many different ones as possible over the week. Use frozen veggies to cut down on waste – when using frozen add 10g to the standard vegetable weight.

Keep tabs on your energy and how long particular combinations of food keep you going. Around half of us find that yoghurt and fruit keeps us going through until lunch, while others find they're hungry again within a couple of hours – seeds or walnuts and apple, or eggs and veg keep them feeling fuller for longer.

> **Cath Weller: I've switched to using 8in (20cm) dinner plates. A smaller portion looks bigger and tricks your brain into thinking you've eaten a bigger meal. I'm very organised and cook for the week ahead at the weekend. Eating like this has forced me to be more creative with my cooking. Now I make vegetable soups. I'll dry roast peppers, tomatoes and onions and bung them all in the oven with cherry tomatoes, then whizz it all down with fresh basil. It makes a beautiful soup. Another favourite is a rainbow slaw which I can add to any protein choices.'**

CALORIES (& SABOTEURS)

Sadly, you are almost bound to come across well-meaning friends or relatives who try to talk you out of what you're doing with HBD – we hear about it time and again. Please be warned. Even though they haven't read *The Human Being Diet* or checked out the references to the scientific research, they may tell you it's 'faddy' and that what you're doing with HBD is not only unhealthy but might even be dangerous.

One of their favourite targets is the low calorie start to HBD. They will likely tell you you're damaging your health and metabolism by following HBD. The two days of Phase 1 (vegetables only) are very low in calories, and over the following 14 days you're still only eating 700–900 calories a day: it is indeed a short and sharp calorie cut. You *are* on a short-term low-calorie regime, with all the benefits the studies have shown, including reduced inflammation, without ever having to count one.

We're eating fewer calories but we're getting more nutrients – we're feeding our bodies with the essential nutrients that they need for health and vitality.

Another favourite is flagging the 'danger' of removing whole food groups at the beginning of the programme: nightshades, dairy and grains. Remember that you're excluding these foods for a short period before reintroducing and taking note of your body's reaction to them. You're excluding them for 16 days as an experiment, to find out whether or not they suit you when they're reintroduced.

You're eating whole fresh foods and every single calorie you're eating is giving you great nutrition. Remember that periods of restricting calories are good for us. If we keep up a low calorie regime for too long, yes, our metabolic rate drops to prevent us from starving. Rest assured that your metabolism isn't going to drop and you won't starve during Reset – you'll just feel better and better each and every day and your body will be forever grateful.

Keep your own counsel and remember you're in this for the long haul. You will achieve your perfect weight by following HBD but you are not on a weight-loss diet. You are eating your way to vibrantly good health. Remind yourself of all the inspiring stories you have heard and the changes, joy and transformation you've seen in your friends.

'To eat is a necessity, but to eat intelligently is an art.'
François de La Rochefoucauld

EATING OUT, HOLIDAYS & WEEKENDS

Remember you need to weigh your food before it's cooked, that it must be cooked without oil, and that you eat just one type of protein per meal. It's easy to navigate holidays and eating out in Phase 3 but not during the Reset. If you do have to attend an event, eat before you go or take your food with you. Most importantly, don't leave the house knowing that you'll be out at lunchtime without taking food with you. Avoid thinking or hoping you'll find an HBD-friendly meal while you're out because in all likelihood you won't. Be as prepared as you possibly can and remember that these 16 days need to be treated as sacrosanct. Set yourself up for success.

Reset weekends can be challenging but there are only two of them. Your first Reset weekend is likely to be easier than the second because you'll be on a high, you'll have jumped in and started to turn your life around. Use your time at weekends to prep and plan and shop for your menu for the following week. Think about batch cooking and freezing a few meals to save you time in the week. Keep busy! As well as prepping and planning your meals, spring cleaning and tidying your cupboards is the order of the day. Keep working on and honing your whys (see page 36).

LIZZIE'S HBD TIPS

Travel
Mass produced, processed and predominantly beige airport and airplane food falls into the 'not worth it' (NWI) category. Who wants to have to start Reset all over again having succumbed to hunger and a soggy croissant filled with plastic cheese? With that in mind, pack a breakfast to eat on the go: your apple plus 35g walnuts or seeds is perfect, or for a main meal, hardboiled eggs or tofu and slaw are great options. Up your water intake and arrive feeling fabulous.

Hotel stays
Start off your day well. Stick to the rules of water on waking and eating within an hour of getting up. The breakfast buffet is your best friend as it is usually laden with seeds, nuts, berries, yoghurt, cheese, eggs and smoked fish – all healthy, delicious and HBD friendly. Remember to take your food scales with you – food weights, especially during Reset, must be 100 percent accurate.

Restaurants
Most restaurants will accommodate your requests – options such as simple, oil-free grilled or steamed fish, or grilled meat or chicken and steamed vegetables are readily available. Many HBDers pop mini bottles of apple cider vinegar into their bag to take with them when they are out and about.

YOUR WHYS

Many people come to HBD because they've witnessed the transformation of friends – seen the weight loss, the energy, the HBD glow and listened to them evangelising about it. But increasingly, more people are turning to HBD to solve other problems – such as aching joints, dodgy bowels, high blood pressure, low mood, lack of energy and unrefreshing sleep. What are *your* whys?

Seasoned HBDers describe their whys as their secret sauce for success. Any time they feel wobbly during the Reset, or fed up or frustrated – especially when friends are out frolicking and having fun at the weekends – they revisit their whys. Reminding yourself of the underlying issues you want to address and change makes the Reset and the whole process more real, more personal and more achievable. Spending this time with yourself, delving into what you want to change and why is a vital part of planning and prepping for success. What was the inspirational dissatisfaction that drew you to HBD? What do you want to change?

Consider distilling what you've written on your phone or in your journal and make a habit of reading it every morning before breakfast. Be really clear with yourself about what you want to change and why it's important to you. How will having glowing skin or a flat stomach, or getting rid of migraine headaches, or achieving your ideal weight make you feel... how will it change your life? Maybe you have a wardrobe full of clothes that are just too small and you're longing to get into them again? Write down how achieving that goal weight will make you feel. Reread your whys and keep them at the forefront of your mind.

> **Amy: 'I just want to say an enormous thank you to you – I'm just reaching Phase 4 of your Human Being Diet and the results for me have been transformative and something I wouldn't have thought possible at the start of this year. I started HBD after reading Cath Weller's article in the *Telegraph* and haven't looked back. I'm 36 and a mum of 3 young children – I was constantly tired, snacking and eating very unhealthily. Now I've lost over 3 stone (19kg) and am just under 8 and a half stone (54kg). I'm between a size 6 and 8, which I still can't quite believe as I was a size 14 when I started HBD. Most importantly, I just feel so much better and happier. I'm reaching the end of Phase 3 now and am determined to keep the weight off. I just felt I had to reach out to say thank you, thank you, thank you!'**

Particularly on days that feel hard – when you're struggling or having a bit of a wobble – keep going back to what you want to achieve and what you want to change with HBD. You are standing on the edge of a new life, of feeling boundless energy, health and joy, and it's time to fly!

HUNKERING DOWN AND RESTING UP

A key piece of advice before you get going is to rest as much as possible during the Reset. You're asking your body to cope with a lot. You'll undergo a deep detox in the first 16 days of HBD – and very often beyond that into Phase 3. We release toxins that are stored in our fat cells (scientifically known as adipocytes if you want to look at some of the research) when we burn fat. When the body is overwhelmed, it pops toxins from our diet (from ultra-processed foods, and pesticide/herbicide residues including glyphosate) into our fat cells and when fat is released from our cells the toxins are too. All this clearing up takes energy!

Early nights are vital for rebalancing and restoring your circadian rhythm – and the importance of sleep just can't be overestimated. It's when we're sleeping that our immune system does its repair work, and it's when we're sleeping that we're burning fat. Nighttime is detoxing time, not just for our body but also for our brain. When we're asleep, toxins and debris that have accumulated during the day are removed by the brain's waste management system. This cleansing and detoxing is vital for brain health and is probably important for protecting against neurodegenerative diseases too.

We all know that feeling of missing out on sleep – we're hungrier and liable to have strong cravings, especially for sugar and carbs, the following day. Your body will thank you for getting early nights and for prioritising sleep (eight hours minimum) throughout the Reset.

On one of your Reset days (thankfully it is normally only one day) typically on day 9, 10, 11 or 12 you might be thinking to yourself: 'I've really had enough of this now, I'm fed up. I feel like throwing in the towel.' This is also normal – remind yourself of that saying, 'It's always darkest before dawn' because it's so true. The other saying I find helpful is: 'Transformation happens on the edge'. Keep going, you can do this – you will be so happy and so proud of yourself for persevering.

Change itself is nearly always uncomfortable – we're creatures of habit. Change not only takes us out of familiar territory and our comfort zone, it also needs energy. But it's all going to be OK! You are going to get through this and the exhilaration, the feeling of elation and pride when you reach day 17, is unimaginably wonderful.

Take it one day at a time and remind yourself that congratulations are in order at the end of every day – we often beat ourselves up for failing – now's the time to congratulate yourself on every day successfully completed. Practise saying to yourself: 'Wow you didn't think you could get through this, but you *did* it, you've done another day – you are incredible and stronger than you ever knew and I'm so proud of you!'

> Remember that when you're preparing and cooking your food, you're showing yourself love and respect. Lay a place setting – and make it look really appealing – as if you were laying the table for someone you love, because you are! And you're showing yourself the love and respect you deserve with this simple act. Aim to eat slowly, take your time and enjoy what you have prepared. This not only gives you more pleasure, it also improves your digestion. Do all you can to avoid eating under stressful or hurried conditions, such as during meetings.

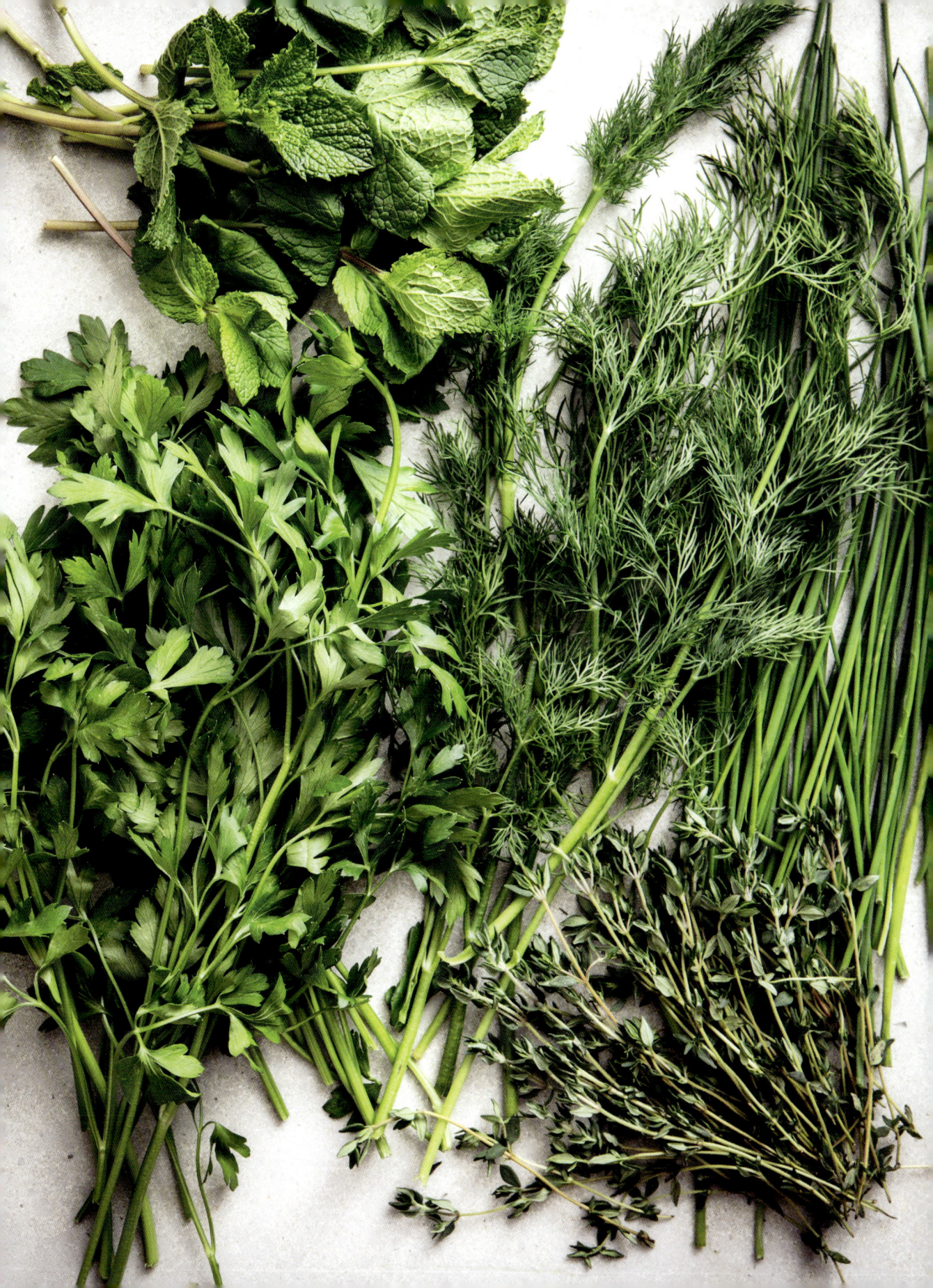

What to Expect

1. How hard will it be?
The first few days can feel hard – you're changing the habits of a lifetime *and* may be experiencing withdrawal and detox effects – see the Detox Tips on page 72 for ways to feel better and remember that the detox effects are temporary and that you'll feel better soon. Many HBDers feel fabulous and absolutely on a high by the end of the Reset, but for some of us the detox continues into Phase 3. Remember, it's a positive sign even when Reset feels difficult.

2. Will I be hungry all the time?
No! After the first two to three days you'll be amazed at how *not* hungry you are, even though you're probably eating less. You're less hungry because your blood sugar is stable and because you are getting the nutrients that you need.

3. What if I make a mistake?
Dust yourself down and just get going again – we nearly all make mistakes when we start something new. But eating sugar or wheat or drinking milk or a glass of wine means starting Phase 2 all over again.

4. Will I have enough energy?
Your energy is likely to be lower than normal for the first few days. Take it easy – go to bed early and get as much rest and sleep as you possibly can. Remember, you're expecting a lot of your body and it's in heavy detox mode. Be patient with yourself and revisit the Detox Tips.

5. How much weight will I lose?
Reset weight loss is often dramatic! A loss of 5–14lb (2.3–6.4kg) is normal but sometimes, depending on how much weight there is to lose, it will be more modest. Even if you're not following HBD for weight loss you are likely to lose a few pounds in Reset. Looking back, when you get to the end of Phase 3, you'll find that weight loss averages out at about 2–3lb (0.9–1.4kg) a week.

6. What if I miss a meal?
It doesn't matter if you don't eat three meals a day in Phase 1. Follow the rules to the letter in Phase 2: make it work for you so you get the results you deserve.

7. What's the most important rule?

All the rules are vitally important, but the number one rule is to read the book *The Human Being Diet* – get to know HBD inside out!

Are you feeling excited about starting? Or would fear be a more accurate word to describe what you're feeling? Psychologists tell us that these two emotions, fear and excitement, are closely connected. I love this quote from Bruce Springsteen's autobiography, *Born to Run*: 'Just before I go on stage, my heart beats a little faster, and my palms sweat, but I know I'm ready. It's not fear – it's excitement. It's my body's way of telling me how deeply I care and how alive I feel.'

It's completely normal to feel apprehensive about starting HBD – nearly everybody does. It's also completely normal to worry about hunger, about your staying power and your willpower. What about those niggling questions in the back of your mind:

'Will this work for me?'

'Will I be the only person for whom HBD doesn't work?'

'Have I wrecked my metabolism by following all those fad diets in the past?'

These are also normal. As long as you read the original book, and read it again, so that you really 'get' the rules and rationale, and as long as you commit – come what may – to getting through this Reset, success is yours. When you're prepping and planning your Reset you are literally planning and prepping for success. Prep like a boss!

HBD does work and it will work for you so long as you follow the rules, as thousands of happy followers have discovered. Keep the faith and trust the process. And trust yourself and prep, prep, prep for success. It doesn't matter what you've tried, or what has or hasn't worked for you in the past – this is different. It's not a weight-loss diet – it's a healthy way of eating and one of the side effects is weight loss. It's not a short term fix – it's a sustainable way of eating, of feasting and fasting, for health, energy and longevity.

This is indeed the most challenging part of the programme and it's also the most important. What you are changing and achieving in the Reset lays a beautiful foundation for success and long-lasting beneficial changes for the rest of your life. The first Reset is definitely the hardest. I promise. Subsequent Resets – the recommendation is one a year – will be a walk in the park. Some HBDers have been in Phase 4 for years without feeling the need for another Reset. It's a personal choice whether you choose to do an annual Reset or not.

HBD Reset Heroes

All fresh whole food contains magical nutrients that support our health – we've picked out a few of the exceptional HBD staples here to inspire you and to illustrate the point that food (and one exercise in particular) really is medicine.

HBD HERO NUMBER 1: WATER – YOUR NEW BEST FRIEND!

If you're feeling hungry, tired or grumpy, water – especially when supplemented with electrolytes – is almost always the answer and comes to the rescue to make you feel better. Fizzy or flat, hot or cold, it doesn't matter as long as it's plain water with nothing added (no lemon juice or cucumber or any other flavouring) except unflavoured, unsweetened electrolytes.

The most important time to drink water is when you wake up in the morning. That's the time you need it most because your immune system has been breaking down fat to energise itself overnight. As mentioned earlier, the fat cells that are broken down contain toxins (when the body can't deal with toxins, it pops them into fat cells to get them out of the way) so early morning water helps to flush out the toxins. Fat isn't just about energy storage but about toxin storage too. Start the day with half a litre of water and drink most of your water (the aim is for 0.35ml per kilo of body weight) before lunch.

You may find that when you start drinking more water you feel thirstier. This is normal – many of those times in the past when you thought you were hungry you were thirsty! Dehydration – lack of water – is recognised as a serious danger to our bodies, which respond by reducing our metabolic rate and our capacity for fat burning. To compensate for the extra water you're drinking, add extra sea salt to your meals and/or supplement with electrolytes.

Tea and coffee don't count towards your water quota and remember that both must be black and unsweetened – and only drunk after or with meals in Phase 2.

HBD HERO NUMBER 2: APPLE CIDER VINEGAR

Apple cider vinegar (ACV) has been used for decades for health and weight loss but there wasn't much scientific evidence to support its use until relatively recently. Studies using 30ml per day have demonstrated the vinegar's powerful effects on blood sugar control, lowering LDL ('bad') cholesterol, decreasing HBA1c and blunting glucose and insulin spikes. It also helps us feel fuller for longer by slowing down the digestion of starchy carbs (think beans and pulses) to sugar. It helps to reduce both sugar and alcohol cravings and lessens bloating too.

Also, the malic acid that apple cider vinegar contains (also found in apples) is antibacterial and antifungal. ACV contains acetic acid, which – wait for it – stimulates GLP-1 hormone, making it a naturally occurring form of GLP-1! As if all that weren't enough, the acetic acid is a short-chain fatty acid that fuels the cells that line our gut – and which also boosts our muscles' uptake of glucose without the exercise!

I hope that's inspired you to try ACV with your meals even if you don't like the idea of it – it's such a powerful health booster and so inexpensive. We are often asked if drinking ACV is harmful to tooth enamel. The answer is that as long as you only have it with meals, either on your salad or diluted in still or sparkling water, it's fine. Organic and unfiltered with 'the mother' is best

Lizzie and I compared notes on our personal preferences for ACV and while we were talking Lizzie told me about a particular brand she didn't like – she described is as slightly acrid and tasting too strong. If you try ACV and don't like it, please don't give up – try another brand; persevere because it's so very good for us.

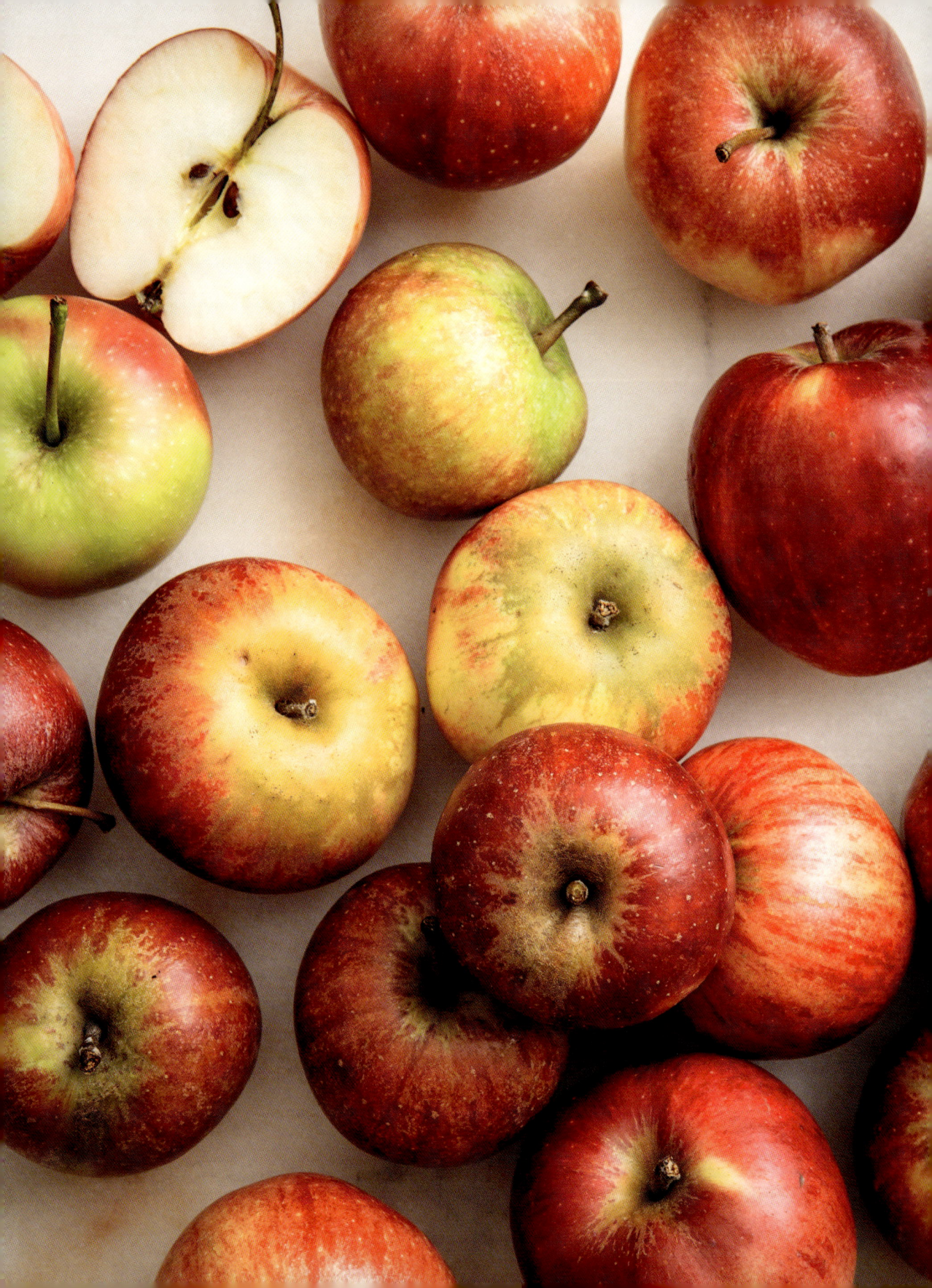

HBD HERO NUMBER 3: APPLE

Much in the way that apple cider vinegar has been used by generations of people for weight loss, and long before scientific evidence was available, the truth of the maxim 'an apple a day keeps the doctor away' has also been proved. Interestingly, years before we had access to the science, we were naturally drawn to the foods and substances that are so good for us.

Some of the key compounds responsible for the apple's health benefits include the antioxidants ursolic acid (UA) and chlorogenic acid (CA) as well as pectin fibre. Both UA and CA have shown effectiveness against fatty liver disease. UA, found in the apple's skin, has the magical ability to improve muscle mass and exercise capacity, along with increasing our levels of brown fat. Brown fat, which is also stimulated by CA, and by fasting and exposure to cold, is a good and helpful fat that burns through our excess stored white fat. It's white fat that's the troublesome kind, bulging over our trousers and wobbling on our bottoms!

Apples also contain plant antioxidants – polyphenols – which protect us against disease and which, along with fibre, nurture our microbiome. So all in all there's a very good chance that an apple a day will keep the doctor away! Eat one apple with or after a meal once a day from Phase 2 onwards. If you're wondering if you can substitute apple juice, even if it's fresh, for an apple, the answer is no! If you juice your apple you're missing out on the wonderful pectin fibre and other compounds it contains. Some of us find, due to a condition known as oral allergy syndrome, that raw apples give us an itchy mouth or throat – if they do that to you try blending or baking them.

HBD HERO NUMBER 4: GREEN VEGGIES

Always the star of the show, greens are rich in fibre, magnesium and other minerals, and plant antioxidants – and they're low in sugar and starch. Include them in your meals every day – show your microbes the love and mix them up. Variety is key. Peas don't count; they're pulses not vegetables! Salad leaves and green herbs definitely do count. Green beans, broccoli, cauliflower (white but an honorary green), cabbage of all colours, artichokes (fresh or bottled in brine), asparagus, courgettes, celery and kale are all great – see the food lists on page 68 for more.

HBD HERO NUMBER 5: AVOCADO

Avocado is a veritable superfood and a delicious source of heart-healthy monounsaturated fats. The maximum amount of avocado allowed per meal in Phase 2 (80g) – has about the same amount of oleic acid as 1 tablespoon of extra virgin olive oil. This is the monounsaturated fat that may lower LDL ('bad') cholesterol. An avocado contains twice as much potassium as a banana and is a great source of fibre.

Filaggrin deficiency (which may be genetic) is associated with dry skin in winter, eczema, alopecia, dermatitis and ichthyosis vulgaris (aka fish skin because it's scaly). Filaggrin is of the utmost importance to skin health for maintaining moisture in the skin, and avocado oil applied topically may help to increase filaggrin production. In clinic I encouraged people who cut an avocado open and found it was brown to slather it on their skin – messy but good for our skin and much better than throwing it away.

Avocado is packed with antioxidants and increases skin firmness and elasticity. Researchers found that eating a small avocado a day for six months improved eyesight and protected older adults from macular degeneration. They're associated with improved cognitive function and brain health too. Wow!

HBD HERO NUMBER 6: OILY FISH

The very best source of omega-3 fats (EPA and DHA) is oily fish. There is no EPA and DHA in plant-based diets apart from in seaweed or algae. Include a portion of oily fish every day – smoked or fresh salmon or mackerel, sardines (in brine or fresh), kippers and herrings. Seabass counts as a semi oily fish – on the omega-3 scale it's about halfway between cod (virtually oil-free) and salmon. Other white fish that are semi-oily include turbot and halibut.

If you're vegan or choose not to eat fish, supplementing with DHA and EPA omega-3 (1–2g per day) with breakfast, is critically important. We need both these omega-3 fats, but most especially DHA, for brain, eye and immune health. We can obtain omega-3s from nuts (especially walnuts) and seeds but we cannot convert them into the meaningful amounts of EPA and DHA we need for good health.

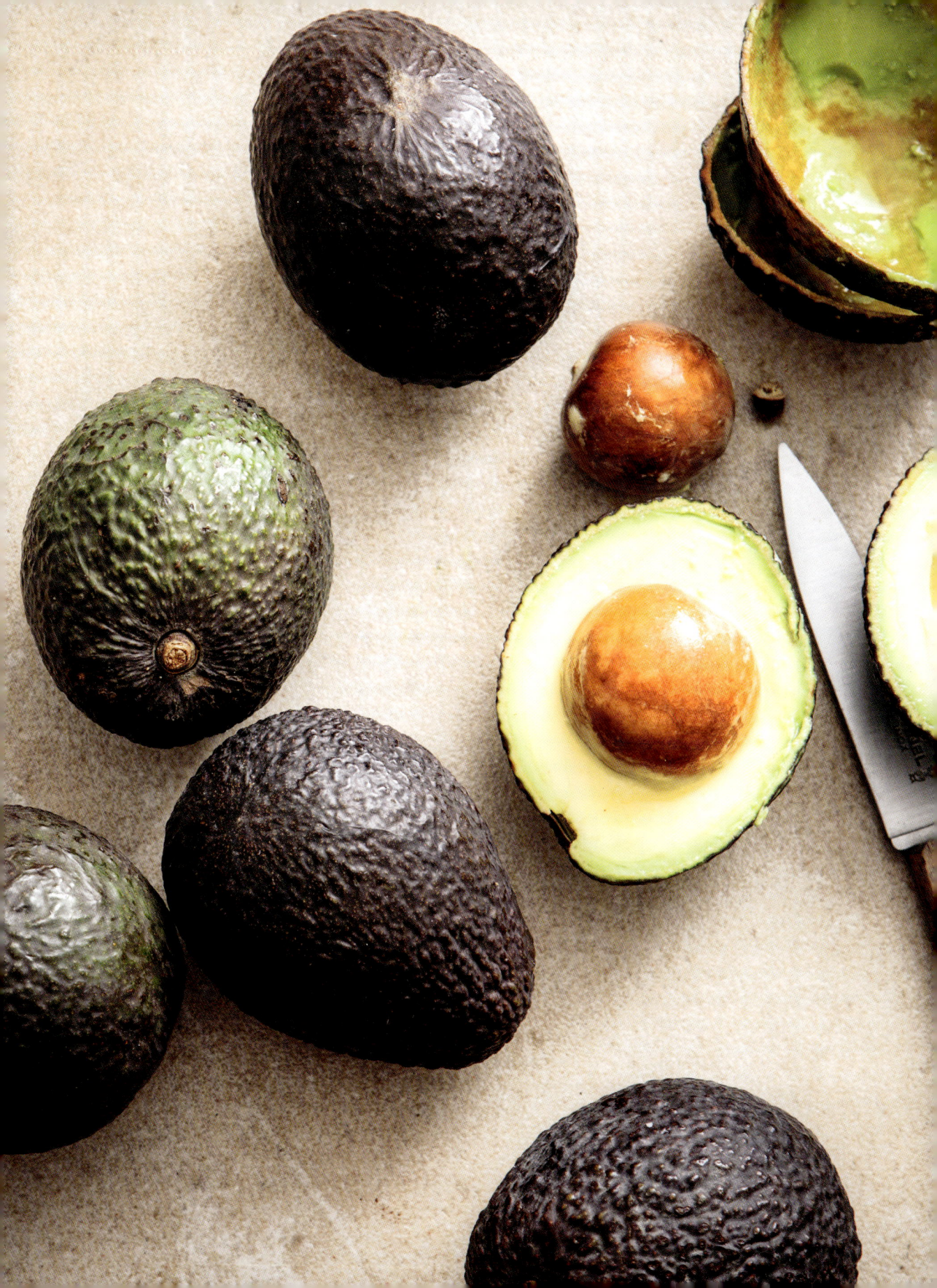

HBD HERO NUMBER 7: PLANT PROTEIN

Protein is all important on HBD – it helps to raise our metabolic rate, keeps us feeling fuller for longer and is vital for maintaining muscle mass. We want to burn fat for energy not our muscles! Protein is key for maximising weight loss. The only high value plant protein is made of soya: tofu and tempeh – eaten in many cultures for millennia.

The most important time to eat protein is within an hour of waking – at breakfast. If you are plant based it's of paramount importance to include tofu (extra firm contains more protein) or tempeh every day to get the protein you need. Textured soy (and mushroom) protein that's made into fake meats and cheese is ultra-processed and is off the menu.

HBD HERO NUMBER 8: WALNUTS

Why are walnuts the only nuts in the HBD? The answer is that they are low in natural sugar, high in healthy fats and much higher in anti-inflammatory omega–3 fats than all other nuts. Scientific research suggests that walnuts have the greatest benefits for heart health and for lowering high blood pressure. And they taste delicious – 35g of walnuts with a chopped or grated apple for breakfast is a quick, easy, delicious and nutritious start to the day. The fibre and fat they contain keeps us going for hours. Activating them is optional; it makes them crunchier and many people find it also makes them easier to digest. If you'd like to try this here's how to do it:

1. Soak the walnuts in filtered water and a little sea salt for 6 hours or longer.
2. Drain and rinse.
3. Spread the nuts on a dehydrator rack or baking tray.
4. Dehydrate in air fryer or very low temperature oven (60°C/140°F/below gas mark 1) for 5 hours or until they are dry and crunchy.
5. Once dried, store in an airtight container.

HBD HERO NUMBER 9: WALKING

Any movement that gets us off our chair and increases the circulation of our blood and lymph (body fluid) is good for us. Walking is the original human exercise! In our caveman days walking was a prerequisite for life itself. Whether we were cold, hungry, thirsty or lonely we took to our feet to find the solution, to find what we needed. In our ancient DNA hunger was a signal to walk, not a signal to open the fridge. Unlike running, or any other intense exercise – which is essentially a stressor and moves us into fight or flight – walking pops us safely back into the parasympathetic nervous system, where we should spend nearly all our time: the place for resting, repairing, regenerating and digesting.

Research suggests that walking in fresh air not only improves our microbiome by increasing microbial diversity but also reduces cortisol and increases stomach acid, which we need for good digestion. The rhythm and regular cadence of a good walk, even if it's just for 10 minutes – and ideally before eating – improves our mood and health. How fast? Fast enough to energise you, but not so fast that you can't hold a conversation without panting. In Reset, gentle walking trumps power walking all the way.

JOURNALLING

The Reset is a fasting and detoxing period. Make time for sitting with yourself, by yourself to deal with feelings and emotions as they surface. Be prepared to feel emotional; it's absolutely normal and it's part of the healing process. In the past, we might have looked to food to change the way we felt. Whether we were bored, sad, anxious, lonely or angry, we literally stuffed those feelings back down and swallowed them as food. But now we must face the feelings head on as they resurface and we need to spend time alone for this. We need to process the feelings, and one of the best ways to do that is not by eating, but by journalling. See James Pennebaker's and John Sarno's powerful work for help with this. *The HBD Journal* is a really useful tool.

LIZZIE'S HBD PANTRY, FRIDGE AND FREEZER STAPLES

INGREDIENTS

Stock up on these staples so you always have the ingredients for delicious HBD meals to hand.

Pantry

- Apple cider vinegar with mother (ACV)
- Colman's English mustard powder or similar
- Tamari (gluten-free soy sauce)
- Dried ground spices and herbs, e.g. dried mixed herbs, ground white pepper, ginger, cumin, coriander, Ceylon cinnamon, nutmeg, paprika*, smoked paprika*, turmeric, chilli, Chinese 5 spice (always check labels for additives – all available online)
- Walnuts
- Sunflower and pumpkin seeds
- Canned, bottled (Bold Bean Co pulses are excellent) or dried chickpeas, butter beans and lentils
- Canned fish in spring water or brine, including tuna, mackerel and sardines
- Coffee and tea
- Sparkling water

STOCKS

There are some excellent fresh stocks available in supermarkets, my favourite being Borough Broth. However, buying fresh stock can be expensive, especially as we use stock in place of oil during Reset and many of us choose to have plenty of soups and broths in Phase 1.

Homemade stock is economical and very satisfying to make. For me, the process of making fresh stock has become a bit of a ritual, an important part of getting my head in the game before I start my annual Reset. It is relaxing and makes the kitchen smell fragrant and wholesome. Pottering in the kitchen and making a batch of stock is the first step into the Reset zone of nourishment and self-care (see recipes on pages 62–63).

Fridge

- Apples, lemons, fresh vegetables (refer to food lists on page 68) salad
- Fresh vegetable and chicken stock (Freja, Borough, Kettle & Fire; always read the labels)
- Fresh herbs and fresh garlic, fresh ginger, fresh chillies*
- Full-fat Greek yoghurt (with dairy proviso)
- Eggs
- Cheese (with dairy proviso) – check labels; no dodgy, lengthy or unpronounceable ingredients!
- Tofu and tempeh (organic)

Freezer

- Frozen berries (one type only, not mixed berry bags)
- Frozen cherries
- Frozen vegetables, including cauliflower rice
- Frozen fish, including salmon and seabass
- Frozen prawns
- Frozen mince, e.g. beef, turkey or chicken, and chicken breasts

Desirables: HBD friendly foods and ingredients beloved by the HBD community

- Flavoured salts including garlic, onion, celery and rosemary salt
- Black garlic, smoked garlic
- Lentil and chickpea rice and pasta (e.g. Mr Organic) – check labels; product must be 100 percent lentil or chickpea
- Red lentil spaghetti (e.g. Profusion, Biona); product must be 100 percent red lentil with no other ingredients
- Gram flour/chickpea flour
- Activated walnuts
- Truffle dust and truffle salt (e.g.Truffle Hunter, Truff or Truffle Guys)
- Vanilla pods, vanilla powder

* contain nightshades

Having a stash of HBD friendly stocks and condiments really helped me to stay on track when I embarked on my first Reset.

Before HBD I was the condiment queen, with a fridge full of sauces, dressings and jellies, most of which, it turned out, were packed with sugar and preservatives. Nevertheless, I love the convenience of condiments and the way a spoonful or two elevates even the simplest of dishes instantly.

Red Pepper Ketchup (see page 56) was dreamt up as an alternative to tomato ketchup. I love Spanish flavours – smoky paprika, sweet peppers and mellow garlic are a dreamy combination. The ketchup is versatile enough to be squeezed on to a burger or tossed through pasta as an impromptu pasta sauce. Once it was created I was hooked (and still am). However, it dawned on me that not all people can eat nightshades and consequently some wouldn't be able to enjoy my pepper ketchup. With that in mind I began casting around for other ideas and inspiration for a series of HBD condiments, seasonings and dressings, many of which have been adapted to be HBD friendly from day 1 of Reset.

Each condiment in the recipes on pages 56–61 has its own identity and place at my table.

HBD EQUIPMENT

- *Potato peeler or mandolin*
- *Nutribullet or food blender*
- *Electric chopper*
- *Good sharp knives*
- *Steamer*

High-quality, non-toxic, non-stick pan
A good-quality non-stick, non-toxic pan will become your best friend. There are ceramic pans available that revolutionise cooking during Reset as they allow you to sear and fry food without using oil. The mini Always pan from Our Place is ideal; it's the perfect size, comes with a lid and can be used on the hob or in the oven.

Bake-O-Glide
If your budget doesn't quite stretch to the Always pan, then invest in a roll of Bake-O-Glide. It is a non-stick, reusable liner that can be cut to size. You can use it to line frying pans and baking sheets.

Air fryer
Air frying allows you to create meals with crisp and crunch and without oil, and is therefore ideal for HBD Phase 2. Fish is delicious cooked in an air fryer: try salmon, bass or bream fillets cooked skin side up and sprinkled with sea salt and spices. The skin crisps up while the flesh stays juicy. You can cook fish fillets on high for about 7–9 minutes (depending on their size) for a perfect speedy and crisp lunch or supper.

Condiments & Stocks

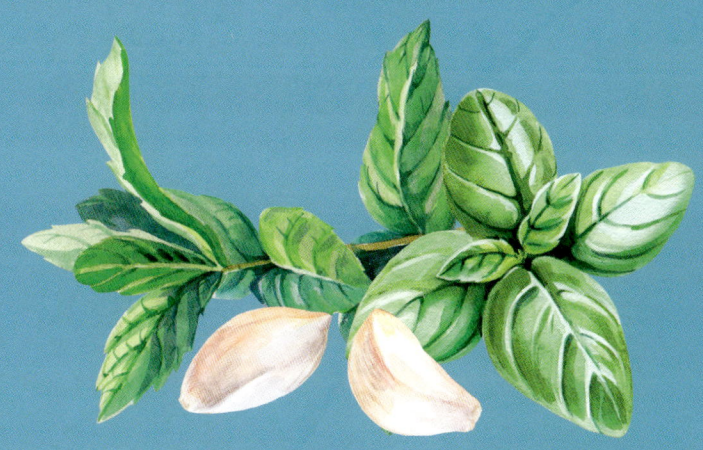

PHASE 1 & 2

RED PEPPER KETCHUP

An HBD staple, this recipe was inspired by the Spanish Rojo Mojo, which quite simply means red sauce. This ketchup is a game-changer: slightly smoky from the paprika, naturally sweet from the roasted peppers – and with a gentle chilli kick. Use it as a condiment, drizzle on fish or chicken, stir through vegetable noodles or add to soups and risottos. An easy way to give simple food a major flavour glow up! This recipe makes 24 tablespoon servings. One tablespoon counts as 15g of your vegetable allowance. This recipe is not suitable for those avoiding nightshades.

PREP: 10 MINUTES
COOK: 50 MINUTES

360g red peppers*, deseeded and quartered
4 garlic cloves, peeled and roughly chopped
1 heaped tsp smoked paprika*
½ tsp chilli powder*
1 tsp apple cider vinegar
sea salt and freshly ground black pepper

1. Preheat the oven to 180°C /160°C fan/gas mark 4.
2. Lay the pepper pieces skin side down in a roasting dish and dot with the chopped garlic. Sprinkle with the spices, a generous grind of salt and pepper and cover tightly with foil. Roast in the oven for 40–50 minutes until tender.
3. Blitz the roasted peppers with the apple cider vinegar until very smooth. Be sure to include all the garlicky, spicy cooking juices from the roasting dish.
4. Keep in a sealed jar in the fridge for up to a week.

TIP: Feel free to add more chilli to taste. For an authentic Spanish twist, try adding some saffron strands when you blitz the sauce. This is fantastic with king prawns and a green salad.

PHASE 2

CHIMICHURRI DRESSING

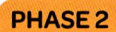

This punchy green Argentine classic is a total HBD winner. Fresh herbs are key – as well as tasting delicious, they keep your microbiome happy. Stir through vegetables in Phase 1. Spoon over a chargrilled steak, pulses or a fish or chicken fillet in Phase 2.

PREP: 10 MINUTES

50g fresh parsley
20g fresh coriander
20g fresh chives
10g fresh mint
½ fresh red chilli* (optional)
2 garlic cloves, peeled and crushed
zest and juice of ½ unwaxed lemon
3 tbsp apple cider vinegar
2 tbsp cold water
1 tsp paprika* (optional)
sea salt and freshly ground black pepper

1. Finely chop all the fresh herbs and the chilli (if using).
2. In a bowl, combine the crushed garlic, lemon zest and juice, the apple cider vinegar, water and paprika (if using). Season generously with salt and pepper and whisk.
3. Add to the fresh herbs and chilli, decant into a jar with a lid and shake.
4. Keeps in the fridge for up to 5 days.

VARIATIONS
- If you are avoiding nightshades you can replace the chilli and paprika with white pepper.

TIP: *Feel free to experiment! Capers add a salty kick, or you could swap these herbs for your favourites. Rosemary and oregano are also delicious with lamb and beef.*

PHASE 1 & 2

PISTOU

Pistou is the French version of pesto, pungent with garlic and basil and a brilliant addition to the HBD condiment repertoire. It's useful to have a jar in the fridge so you can add a spoonful as a seasoning to soups and stews or drizzle on salads or over pasta. Pistou provides an instant flavour glow up for many simple dishes. Purists may object, but I adore the combination of lemon and basil – and love the addition of lemon zest in Phase 2 and beyond.

PREP: 10 MINUTES

100g fresh basil
2 garlic cloves, sliced
1 tsp lemon zest
   (for Phase 2 onwards)
sea salt and freshly ground
   white pepper

TIP: *Blanching the basil before combining it with the other ingredients helps to preserve its vibrant green colour.*

1. First blanch the basil. Bring a saucepan of water to the boil, add the basil and leave for about 5 seconds, strain and immediately transfer the basil to a bowl of iced water to stop the cooking process.
2. Put the basil, garlic, a pinch each of salt and white pepper and the lemon zest (if using) into a blender. Add a splash of cold water and blend thoroughly, adding more water if necessary until the pistou comes together and has a pouring consistency. It can take up to a minute to ensure the ingredients are fully amalgamated, so be patient.
3. Store for up to 3 days in a small jar in the fridge or freeze immediately in an ice cube tray. The frozen cubes can be added to soups and stews directly from the freezer or quickly defrosted if used on pasta or salads.

PHASE 1 & 2

MUSTARD DRESSING

Having a jar of tangy, garlicky dressing in your fridge is a must in my opinion. This is an easy and delicious way to give a simple salad an instant glow up during Reset. Adding great flavour to your food doesn't need to be complicated: punchy mustard, garlic and apple cider vinegar do the trick perfectly. This is also brilliant drizzled over grilled Mediterranean vegetables or served 70s style in half an avocado.

PREP: 5 MINUTES

2 tbsp cold water
2 tbsp apple cider vinegar
1 small garlic clove, crushed
2 level tsp English mustard powder
generous pinch of sea salt and freshly ground black pepper

1. Whisk all the ingredients together thoroughly.
2. Use immediately or decant into a clean jar and refrigerate. It will keep for up to a week in the fridge, but remember to shake vigorously before use.

TIP: *You can choose to add fresh soft herbs. A tarragon vinaigrette is delicious with cold chicken. Chives or dill are great additions for cold poached salmon or smoked salmon salads.*

PHASE 1 & 2

CURRY SAUCE

I was inspired to create an HBD chip shop curry sauce after a visit to The Mayfair chippy whose curry sauce is arguably the best in London. Just a few simple ingredients combine to make a sweet and fruity sauce with a gentle curry kick. I like the addition of ginger, which brings depth of flavour and interest; however, if you're after a more authentic chip shop taste, then leave it out. This is brilliant with fish in Phase 2 and sweet potato fries in Phase 3, and an easy way to pimp up a plain chicken breast or grilled steak. If you're a fan of curry, I urge you to give it a go. About 1 tablespoon is 15g of your vegetable allowance in Phase 2.

PREP: 10 MINUTES
COOK: 45–60 MINUTES

1 small butternut squash, unpeeled, halved and deseeded
2 tsp mild curry powder
1 tsp turmeric
1 tsp ground coriander
½ tsp ground cumin
½ tsp grated fresh ginger (optional)
boiling water
sea salt and freshly ground black pepper

TIP: *Freeze in ice cube trays to defrost quickly when required.*

1. Preheat the oven to 190°C /170°C fan/ gas mark 5.
2. Place the butternut squash flesh side up in a deep roasting dish with a splash of cold water (so the squash steams slightly as it roasts) and a generous grind of salt and pepper. Cover tightly with foil and roast for 45–60 minutes, depending on the size of the squash (it should be soft).
3. Allow to cool slightly before scooping the flesh into a blender and discarding the skin.
4. Put the curry powder, turmeric, ground coriander and cumin into a small non-stick pan and gently dry fry to release their aromas.
5. Add the warm spices, ginger, a grind of salt and pepper and a splash of freshly boiled water to the blender with the squash.
6. Blitz until silky, adding splashes of boiling water until you have a sauce with the consistency of tomato purée.
7. Keeps in a sealed jar in the fridge for up to 5 days or freezes well.

VARIATION
- Add 3–4 tablespoons to meat or pulses, stock and vegetables for a quick midweek curry.

PHASE 2

MANGO CHUTNEY

Sticky, sweet and packed with fragrant spices, this mango chutney is deliciously moreish. It is simple to prepare and a wonderful treat to have in the fridge, ready to be slathered on almost anything. It's delicious with curries or bhajis and exceptionally good with a strong, mature Cheddar or with grilled chicken. Feel free to dial up the chilli for added fire and spice. These quantities make 4 portions; deduct 10g from your veggie allowance per serving. It counts as your fruit for a meal. The chutney will keep in the fridge for 2–3 days and freezes well.

PREP: 10 MINUTES
COOK: 25 MINUTES

80g onion, finely chopped
100ml cold water
6 cardamom pods, seeds removed and crushed
¼ tsp ground coriander
¼ tsp nigella seeds
1 garlic clove, finely chopped
400g fresh mango, chopped
1 tsp tamari
2 tsp apple cider vinegar
½ tsp sea salt
1 tsp grated fresh ginger
1 small, fresh mild chilli*, finely chopped (optional)

1. In a small pan, simmer the onion in the water over a medium heat until softened, about 5–7 minutes.
2. In a separate pan, gently warm the crushed cardamom seeds, ground coriander and nigella seeds for 1–2 minutes to release their flavour and aroma.
3. Add the garlic, mango, tamari and apple cider vinegar to the softened onion. Cover the pan with a lid and simmer until the mango has softened and broken down – about 8–10 minutes. Stir regularly and use the back of a wooden spoon to further break up the softened mango pieces.
4. Add the sea salt, cardamom, coriander, nigella seeds, ginger and chilli, if using. Continue to cook uncovered over a low heat until the chutney becomes syrupy and the water has evaporated – about 4–5 minutes.
5. Allow to cool completely. Store in an airtight container in the fridge.

PHASE 1 & 2

THE BEST CHICKEN BONE STOCK

Maximising flavour is the secret of a fabulous stock. Roasting the chicken bones or wings with herbs and vegetables until they are burnished and sticky takes the flavour of the stock to the next level. Simmering the bones releases all the precious collagen, so you are left with an ambrosial stock, packed with flavour and nutrients – an amazing base for so many recipes.

PREP: 15 MINUTES
COOK: 2.5 HOURS

500g chicken bones or chicken wings
2 onions, quartered
5 garlic cloves, whole, unpeeled
2 large carrots, washed and roughly chopped
1 leek, washed and roughly chopped
1 stick of celery, roughly chopped
2 bay leaves
1 tsp black peppercorns
2 sprigs of thyme and rosemary
2 litres boiling water
sea salt and freshly ground black pepper

1. Preheat the oven to 180°C/160°C fan/gas mark 4.
2. Spread the chicken bones or wings, the onions, garlic, carrots, leek, celery, bay leaves, peppercorns, thyme and rosemary on a deep roasting tray and season with salt and pepper.
3. Add cold water to cover the base of the roasting tray to a depth of about 1cm. Roast uncovered for 30 minutes until everything is caramelised and the water has evaporated. Remove the tray from the oven and transfer the chicken bones and vegetables to a large saucepan.
4. Deglaze the roasting tray with a little boiling water, using a wooden spoon to scrape up the sticky residue; this will add colour and flavour to the stock. Add this, along with the remaining boiling water, to the saucepan. Simmer for a minimum of 2 hours or longer, topping up with a little extra boiling water if necessary.
5. Sieve into a clean jar and refrigerate. When the stock is chilled, it will become gelatinous due to the high collagen content. A thin layer of fat and sediment will form on the surface; remove this with a metal spoon before use.
6. The stock will stay fresh for up to 5 days in the fridge or can be frozen.

TIP: I have used chicken wings here as they are readily available and inexpensive. Many butchers sell fresh chicken bones, which also work well. Alternatively, use bones left over from a roast chicken. Simply carve the meat and immediately roast the bones as above.

PHASE 1 & 2

CLASSIC VEGETABLE STOCK

A good veggie stock is invaluable for cooking in Phase 2 and for making stews and soups. I like to keep it simple, using scrubbed organic veggies, fresh herbs and spices. Unlike bone broth, you don't need to simmer this stock for hours, as that would result in an acrid taste.

PREP: 10 MINUTES
COOK: 1 HOUR

2 onions, quartered
1 head of garlic, unpeeled and washed, halved horizontally
2 large carrots, washed and roughly chopped
1 leek, washed and roughly chopped
1 stick of celery, roughly chopped
2 bay leaves
1 tsp black peppercorns
2 sprigs each of fresh thyme, rosemary and parsley
1.5 litres freshly boiled water
generous pinch of sea salt

1. Place all the ingredients in a large saucepan and cover with the freshly boiled water. Simmer uncovered for 1 hour.
2. Pour through a sieve into a clean jar and refrigerate. Keep in the fridge for up to 5 days or freeze.

TIPS: *Feel free to play with the flavours by adding different herbs and spices.*
The stock can be made using veggie trimmings; be sure to wash them first.

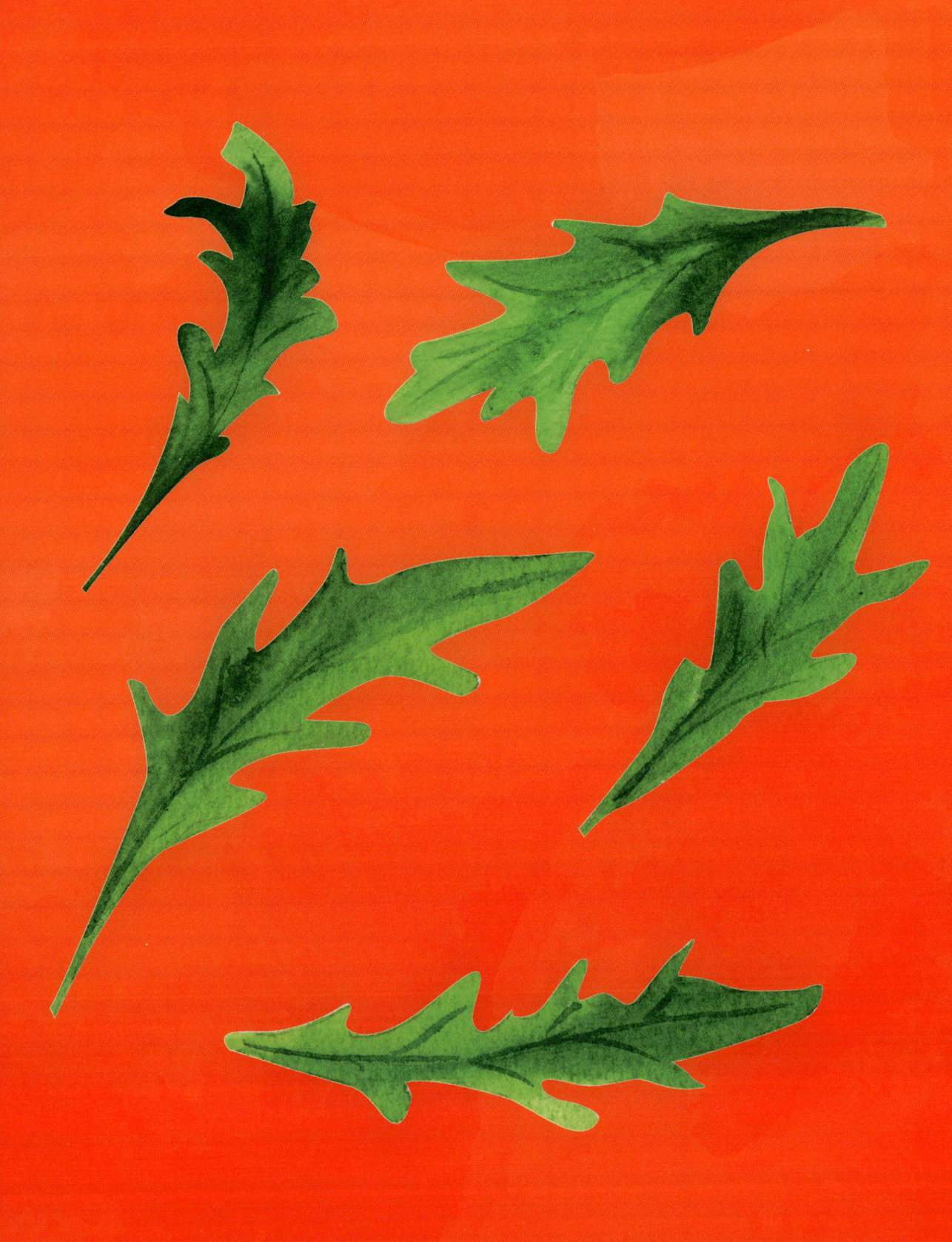

PHASE 1

The Reset Rules
– we're getting
ready to start!

PHASE 1 – IT'S ALL ABOUT THE VEG

This is a two-day vegetable fast, which means no oil, alcohol, sugar, honey or sweeteners. No dairy, protein foods or pulses and no fruit or grains. Just vegetables! Your vegetables can be made into soup using clear, liquid vegetable or chicken stock, which can be homemade – see Lizzie's recipes – or bought at a supermarket (always check labels – see page 69). Vegetables provide minerals and wonderful fibre, which is not only beloved by our friendly microbes, but which also helps to keep us feeling fuller for longer. Vegetable fibre, like tiny scrubbing brushes, cleans and detoxes our intestines. There are no weight limits for foods in Phase 1 but once you move into Phase 2 food weights are all important.

1. Only eat the foods on the list.

2. Vegetables only for two days!

3. Black and unsweetened coffee/tea/green tea/herbal tea can be drunk freely through the day. No fruit teas.

4. Drink lots of water – fizzy or flat, hot or cold – to help you detoxify and to energise you.

5. Remember, no fruit – not even an apple – until day three!

You will see that the Phase 1 veg list includes nightshades. Nightshades are only included for seasoned HBDers who are doing their annual reset and who know that nightshades suit them. See Potentially Problematic Foods (see pages 32–33) to find out why. If a food is not listed, it's not allowed.

GET READY

Preparation is key: most people struggle if they don't have the right tools for the job and HBD is no different. The more HBD store cupboard staples and prepared meals you have to hand the easier and more enjoyable your Reset will be.

A good fresh stock is crucial, either shop bought or homemade. It's used in place of oil during Reset and is the basis for many soups, broths and stews. Freezing fresh stock in ice cube trays is a great idea; these little cubes are your substitute for oil or stock cubes for the next 16 days. You can use them straight from the freezer, melt them in a pan and start cooking.

As part of your preparation make a big box of slaw, or a chopped salad, to keep in the fridge ready for you to dig into when hunger strikes. The five hour fast between meals rule doesn't apply until you move into Phase 2. Soups and broths are my own personal Reset heroes. I find it helps enormously to be able to reach for a warm mug of soup when I feel tired or hungry in Phase 1.

The joy of Phase 1 is that there is no need to fast: it is one time in HBD you are allowed to nibble whenever you choose to, so I urge you to make the most of it. Whether homemade cups of soup, salads or simple steamed vegetables or crudites, enjoy the freedom of being able to eat when you want.

LIZZIE'S HBD TIPS

Welcome to the first day of the rest of your life! You'll never regret taking this step forward and embracing the magic that HBD will bring to your sense of well-being and vibrant health.

That said, this can be a time of mixed emotions: there can be fear of the unknown, fear of hunger and ultimately fear of failure. It's normal to experience intense emotions – I certainly did – but rest assured those feelings do pass if you just take it one day at a time. As the world's greediest foodie, I promise that if I can do it, then so can you.

Phase 1 really needn't be 48 hours of hunger and deprivation. Reframe it as an opportunity to rest, calm your digestive system and nourish your body with fragrant soups, broths, salads and veggie stews. The Reset is the perfect excuse to check out of the hurly burly of life and concentrate on self-care and replenishing your body and soul.

This chapter is full of recipes, inspiration and tips to help you navigate the first 48 hours of your HBD adventure. It offers simple ways to transform fresh vegetables and include more herbs and spices in your diet. Coupled with some new, simple cooking techniques, it will help you breeze through Phase 1.

PHASE 1 FOOD LIST – IF IT'S NOT LISTED IT'S NOT ALLOWED!

Approximately 500g of vegetables per meal as a guideline

Aim to eat at least 3 different vegetables in every meal

Vegetables	
Artichokes (fresh or bottled in brine)	Kohlrabi
Asparagus	Leeks
Aubergines*	Lettuce (all types, including iceberg, romaine, lamb's lettuce)
Avocados	
Broccoli	Mushrooms
Brussels sprouts	Okra
Butternut squash	Olives (max 4 per meal)
Cabbages	Onions
Capers (in brine and sugar-free)	Pak choi
Carrots	Peppers*
Cauliflower	Radishes
Celery	Rocket
Chicory	Romanesco
Chinese leaf lettuce	Salsify
Courgettes	Samphire
Cress	Sauerkraut
Cucumber	Seaweed
Endive	Shallots
Fennel	Spring greens
Gherkins or dill pickles (sugar-free)	Spring onions
Green beans	Spinach
Kale	Tomatoes*
Kimchi*	

*denotes nightshade

*Nightshade vegetables are marked with an asterisk. Recipes that include nightshade vegetables are marked with 🌙.

Phase 1 optional extras	
Black coffee Black/green/white tea Herbal tea	Can be drunk freely throughout both days. No added milk of any kind and no sugar or sweeteners. No fruit teas.
Seasoning	Any fresh, dried, frozen herbs and spices including chilli*, garlic, ginger, turmeric, sea salt, Himalayan salt, black and white pepper. Ensure there are no additives in mixed seasonings and herb packets.
Apple cider vinegar	Unpasteurised and organic with 'the mother'. Add to food or mix in water to drink with meals.
Clear liquid vegetable stock (no stock cubes or bouillon powder)	Waitrose, Planet Organic, Whole Foods, Borough, Freja.

*denotes nightshade

No sweetcorn or peas – they are not vegetables! No potatoes or sweet potatoes! Why no bouillon or stock cubes? Here are the ingredients in a typical vegetable stock cube: salt, vegetable fats (palm, shea, sal butter), potato starch, yeast extract, sugar, onion powder, carrots, herbs, spices, tomato powder, red pepper, caramel syrup, flavourings, leek, maltodextrin.

We don't want added sugars, fats or artificial flavourings that have been conjured up in a lab. Here are the ingredients in Borough Chicken Bone Broth (this one is organic and is Lizzie's favourite ready-made stock) ingredients: spring water, chicken bones (40%), carrots, onions, apple cider vinegar, black peppercorns, pink Himalayan salt, thyme, bay leaves. Perfect!

Freja Instant Bone Broth is off limits because of the ingredients highlighted in bold: chicken bone broth powder (61%), **yeast extract (yeast extract, salt)**, tomato powder*, **natural flavouring**, sea salt, **olive oil,** ground thyme, garlic powder, onion powder, ground white pepper. But Freja Chicken Bone Broth Protein is fine – ingredients: free-range chicken bone broth.

Some of these ingredients serve as useful reminders: reading food labels is all important. Watch out for and avoid 'natural flavours', sugar and added oil or fat. When you start Phase 2 you might be amazed to see sugar included on the labels of foods such as smoked salmon and cooked prawns. Always, always check labels – it's a great new habit to get into.

DAY 1 PHASE 1 – EPSOM SALTS

It's recommended, but not a rule, to take three teaspoons of Epsom salts dissolved in water on the first day of Phase 1. Take them 30 minutes or longer before breakfast. They taste awful but you should only need to take them once. Stir to dissolve them in half a cup of hot water, add cold water and drink. Then drink more water to take the taste away. The salts act as a laxative to clear out your gut, which helps to minimise detox symptoms.

Epsom salts, which are not salt at all but magnesium, have long been used by naturopaths for patients suffering from constipation and/or gallbladder problems, including gallstones. The salts increase bile flow and dilate the bile ducts, which allows gallstones to be expelled. I, and most seasoned HBDers, take the three teaspoons of Epsom salts recommended on the first day of the Reset.

Be warned that the salts can result in a dramatic evacuation, but everyone reacts to them differently. Stay at home! You definitely don't want to take them before setting off on the school run or your commute. Happily, the worst is normally over by lunchtime. Any Epsom salts, as long as they are 100 percent magnesium sulphate with no additives, will do fine. If nothing happens after the first dose, repeat it before breakfast on day two. It's rare, but occasionally they just don't work – don't worry if that's the case, just keep going with the programme.

If you're scared or feel uneasy about taking them, don't take them! If you are in any doubt about their safety because of something you've heard or read on the internet, do not take them without first consulting your doctor. Avoid Epsom salts and all supplements if you have kidney disease. Consult your doctor if you are taking prescription medication before taking any supplements, including Epsom salts.

Some people breeze through Phase 1 and others find it challenging, but remember, it only lasts two days and you have the luxury of protein to look forward to on day three. Keep drinking the water! And reframe any feelings of discomfort into positive thoughts: 'this is just what my body needs – I've been dreaming of a detox and turning over a new leaf and this is what it feels like! I know it won't last for long but this is a sign that I really needed to do this and I'm proud of myself for getting through it.'

LIZZIE'S HBD TIPS

In an ideal world you would embark on your Reset when there is a lull in the to-ing and fro-ing of life events – when your world is peaceful and calm, allowing you time to rest and rejuvenate and focus on yourself. For those of us with large families, however, it's not always straightforward! Creating separate meals is hard work – it means twice the planning, twice the shopping and twice the cooking. At the same time it's unrealistic and inappropriate to expect the whole family to join you in the Reset. I know that this would have resulted in riots at my place with my hungry, growing teenagers.

To avoid family uproar and to minimise extra work, we've created HBD workarounds. The solution is in dishes that tick the HBD Reset box and keep everyone happily fed – meals that can be prepared for everyone and adapted slightly to ensure that they are Reset friendly for you.

Crowd-pleasing dishes must be satisfying and delicious – meals that everyone looks forward to eating. Seeing the surprised look on family faces when they realise that they too are eating the HBD way, and it all tastes delicious, is a sign that you have succeeded. This is the key to turning HBD into a forever lifestyle for the whole family.

DETOX OR WITHDRAWAL?

The detox, which for many of us continues through the Reset and into Phase 3, is deep – both physically and emotionally – and can feel pretty tough. But it is profoundly healing. For most first timers the Reset is a massive period of adjustment. Your brain and body have gone cold turkey on many of the foods and drinks they've come to rely on and that have become part of daily life. Everything from cappuccinos to croissants, sugar and biscuits, bread and beer or wine. While many sail through the first 16 days with no ill effects, others find them seriously challenging.

Detox and withdrawal effects can make us feel rough. Some people experience flu-like symptoms with headaches, achiness, brain fog, tearfulness, twitchy or restless legs, sweating, nausea, bowel changes and a nasty taste in the mouth. These symptoms are all normal and happily all short lived. They are proof that something deeply healing is happening below the surface – these detox symptoms are sometimes referred to as a 'herxheimer reaction' or 'healing crisis'.

The detox – tips for feeling better in Reset

- Drink lots of water, to flush out toxins and to provide energy.
- Add sea salt to your water or just put a pinch on your tongue to help with energy.
- Add unsweetened, unflavoured electrolytes to your water to help energise and hydrate you.
- Try hot water in a mug, especially if you're resetting in winter. It is warming and comforting.
- Drink herbal teas freely in Phase 1 but only with meals in Phase 2. No fruit teas.
- Try soup – comfort in a mug. There are delicious Phase 1 soup recipes here.
- Take painkillers – tablets or capsules rather than powders or liquids – if you need to.
- Have hot baths with Epsom salts – see below.
- Use hot water bottles – detoxing can make you feel cold.
- Add layers of clothing – ditto.
- Wear bed socks – ditto.
- Reframe feelings of cold or discomfort: this is what fat-burning feels like and I love it!
- Keep a journal.
- Prioritise hugging! We get oxytocin, that lovely feelgood bonding hormone, when we hug the people and pets we love.
- Go for gentle walks in the fresh air.
- Get as much rest as possible.

Electrolytes are minerals: sodium, potassium, magnesium and chloride, which affect hydration, blood pH and muscle function. Muscle cramps, twitchy legs or feeling light-headed during Reset may be a sign that you need more of some of these minerals which are lost along with excess water from our bodies during the detox. When our insulin levels fall (due to excluding sugar and starchy carbs) we burn glycogen, which is stored sugar, and that makes our kidneys excrete more water.

All electrolytes are minerals but not all minerals are electrolytes. Any unflavoured and unsweetened electrolyte drops will do, e.g. Viridian

Cath Weller in the *Telegraph,* **who lost 3 stone (42kg) with HBD: 'Was I hungry? Yes, you are hungry in the first week until you get used to it and I'm someone who doesn't really like vegetables, so that wasn't easy. But the results were so astonishing, it was incredibly motivating. When something really does work, you want to stick with it. I lost 11lb (5kg) in the first two weeks and I could feel a difference in my health straight away. My gut was less tender and my skin was glowing.'**

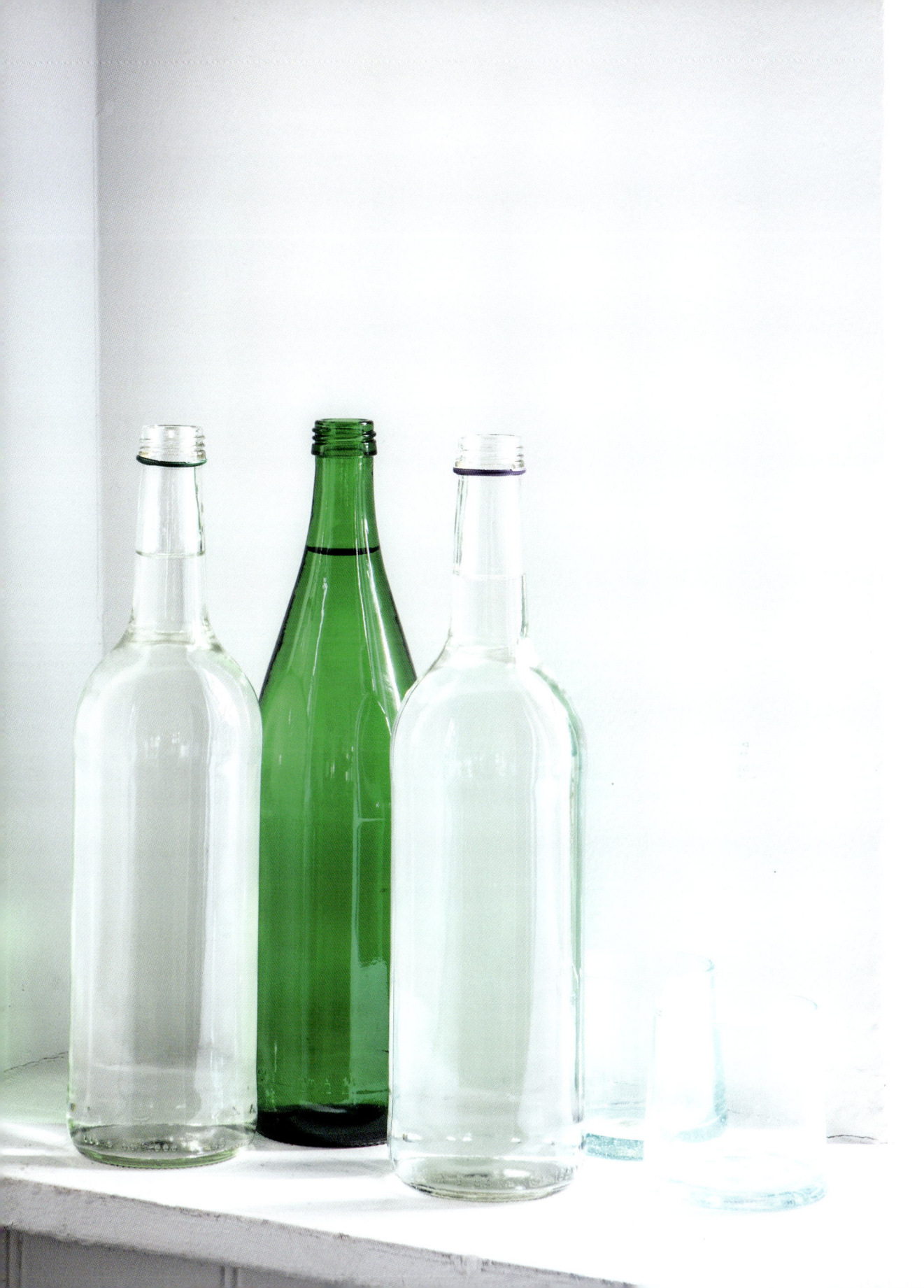

Electrolyte Fix, ConcenTrace, Elete Electrolyte, BodyBio Elyte – they make water taste better too. Many HBDers (myself included) add electrolytes to our water and also supplement with around 400mg magnesium glycinate/bisglycinate every day. Magnesium, which we need more of when we're stressed, is vital for sleep as well as for energy.

Epsom salt baths can have a magical effect, not only for speeding up the detox process but also for deeper, more refreshing sleep. We absorb the magnesium, which is what they're made of, through our skin. Add about 500g to a hot bath, swirl the salts round with your hand to dissolve them and soak for at least 10 minutes – longer, adding hot water as needed, is better. Dry off and hop straight into bed with a book.

Cath Weller in the *Telegraph,* **on keeping the weight off in Phase 4: 'I don't have a lot of time for exercise, but I do take my dog Margot for a 40-minute walk before work and that's when I think and process everything, it's like a form of meditation. Other than that, I do ten minutes of HIIT (high-intensity interval training). I don't eat ready meals or any ultra-processed food. The other major difference is the quantities I eat. I love cheese but now I'll only eat a matchbox-sized 80g piece or three slices of halloumi. I only eat carbs at the weekend as part of a treat meal. I'll also treat myself to the occasional Thai takeaway on the weekend.'**

SLOW DOWN
You are doing something incredible for yourself and for your loved ones. HBD is the ultimate self-care, so support the Reset process by slowing down and making time for yourself whenever you can. Give yourself permission to say no to the demands and stresses of life for 16 short days. Your metamorphosis, a little like a butterfly's, will be nothing short of miraculous!

Checklist

Read *The Human Being Diet* and read it again. Make sure you've spent time working out and writing down your whys. Have you looked at your diary and found 16 clear days – have you chosen a day to start? It's a good idea to begin at a weekend. Remember to plan and plot as though you're doing this for your best friend, making sure that you're laying the foundations for success. Stock your fridge ready for the week ahead. You might find these items helpful to make the reset as successful as possible:

- ☐ Tape measure: measure round your belly button, the widest part of your hips and the widest part of your left leg – write down your measurements. Sometimes the scales don't reflect fat loss but your measurements do!

- ☐ Digital food scales

- ☐ Food containers for meals on the go, including soup flasks

- ☐ Water filter

- ☐ Pint or half litre glass or large water flask

- ☐ Food diary

- ☐ Ceramic non-stick pan

- ☐ Apple cider vinegar with the 'mother'

- ☐ Epsom salts for the first day in Phase 1 (and for adding to your bath)

- ☐ Small plates and bowls (to make your portions look bigger)

- ☐ Score troublesome symptoms weekly out of ten (such as bloating, headaches or joint pain) and witness them lessen and gradually disappear

- ☐ Body scales or a body composition analyser (optional)

PHASE 1

Soups & Main Meals

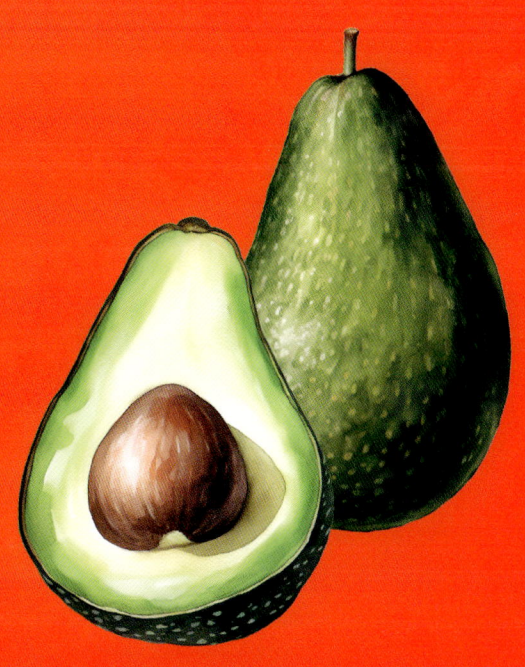

THAI-STYLE RAMEN

This broth feels deeply comforting and healing; it is gently infused with fragrant lemongrass, lime leaves, mellow garlic and warming ginger. Delicate pak choi, meaty shiitake mushrooms and sweet carrot noodles will keep hunger at bay.

SERVES 2
PREP: 10 MINUTES
COOK: 15 MINUTES

400ml fresh chicken or vegetable stock
200ml boiling water
3 garlic cloves, whole, peeled
1 stick of lemongrass, bashed (see Tip)
1 lime leaf
1 thumb-sized piece of ginger, peeled
1 small whole Thai chilli* (optional)
1 carrot, cut into very fine strips (see step 3)
150g shiitake mushrooms, quartered
1 head baby pak choi, roughly chopped
fresh coriander, to serve
sea salt and freshly ground black pepper

1. Put the stock and boiling water into a saucepan. Add the garlic, lemongrass, lime leaf, ginger and chilli (if using). Bring to a very gentle boil and simmer for 2–3 minutes before removing from the heat.
2. Leave for 10 minutes to infuse before straining.
3. Make the carrot strips while the stock infuses. Use a sharp pointed knife to make incisions along the length of the carrot. Shave off very fine ribbons with a potato peeler. Return the infused stock to the saucepan and add the carrot, shiitake mushrooms and a pinch of sea salt. Simmer for 2–3 minutes before adding the pak choi and simmering for a further 1–2 minutes.
4. Taste and adjust the seasoning as needed, adding more salt if required. Serve with fresh coriander.

TIP: *Gently pounding or bashing lemongrass with a rolling pin before cooking allows the stalk to release more flavour.*

VARIATION
- If you are avoiding nightshades, replace the chilli with a pinch of white pepper.

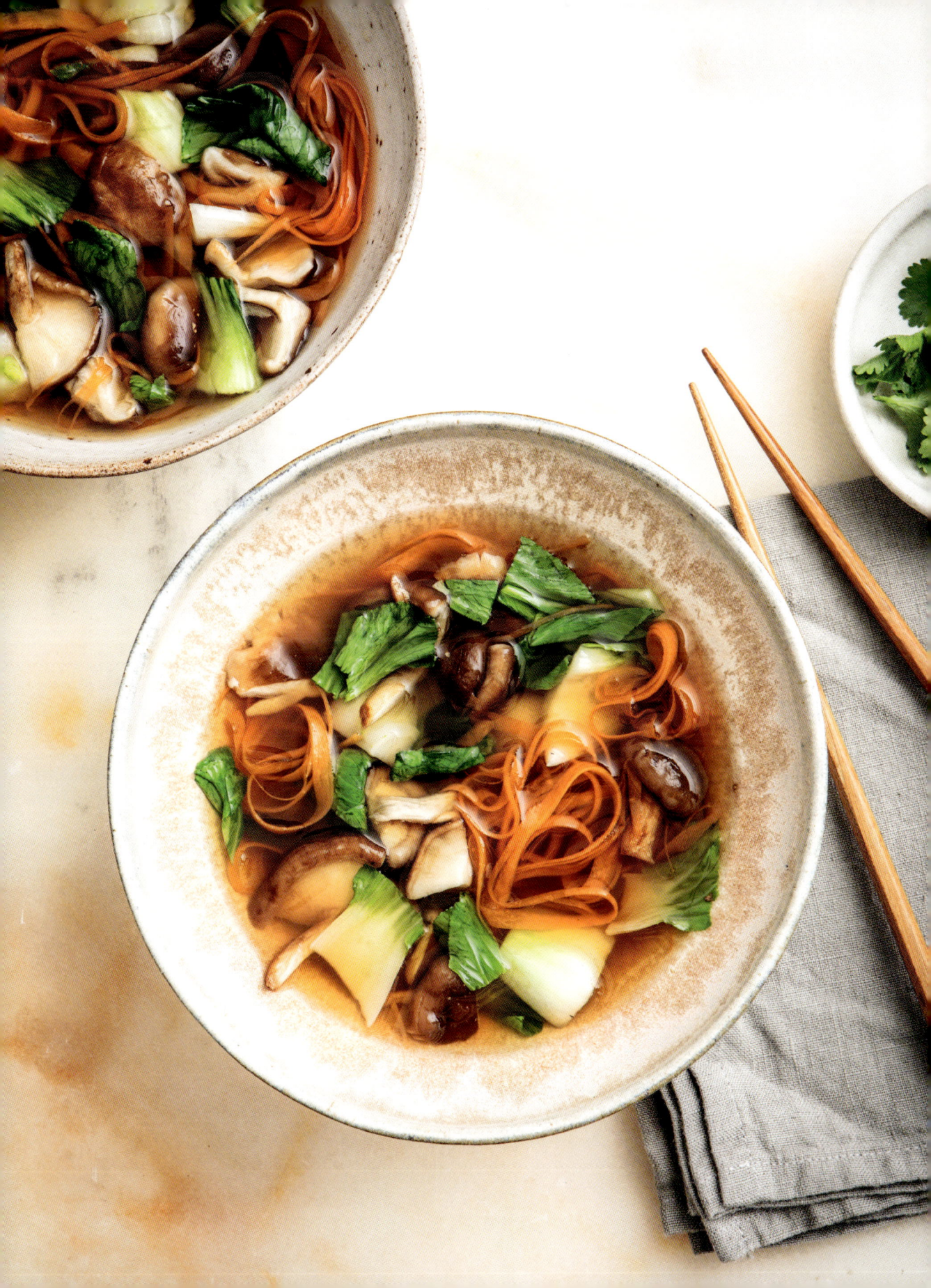

BUTTERNUT SQUASH, TURMERIC & GINGER SOUP

A gloriously fragrant and delicious soup, full of wonderfully healing ingredients. Golden and earthy turmeric, sweet butternut squash and warming fresh ginger are a wonderful flavour combination. This soup is great for both your body and soul as the spices have many nutritional benefits. Turmeric is packed with phytonutrients, while ginger is an antioxidant – and both have anti-inflammatory properties. This soup also freezes well.

SERVES 2–3
PREP: 5 MINUTES
COOK: 25 MINUTES

1 small onion, diced
500ml fresh chicken or vegetable stock
1 large butternut squash, peeled and chopped
3 garlic cloves, chopped
2 fresh tomatoes*, chopped (optional)
1 tsp ground turmeric
1 tsp ground ginger
fresh coriander or chives, to serve
sea salt and freshly ground black pepper

1. In a large saucepan, cook the onion in a splash of the stock until soft. Add the butternut squash, garlic, tomatoes, turmeric, ginger, the remaining stock and a generous pinch of sea salt.
2. Simmer over a low heat for about 15–20 minutes until the butternut squash is soft.
3. Use a hand blender to purée the soup until it is silky smooth. Add a few splashes of boiling water if the soup is too thick.
4. Check the seasoning, adding salt and pepper as necessary and serve with a scattering of fresh herbs.

TIP: *Omit the tomatoes if avoiding nightshades.*

FRENCH ONION & THYME SOUP

One of my all-time favourites; mellow, sweet, caramelised onions roasted in stock, thyme and garlic. Dry frying the onions releases their natural sugars, which then catch and caramelise slightly as they cook. It is this process that gives the soup such depth of flavour and a deep amber colour. The soup freezes well.

SERVES 2
PREP: 10 MINUTES
COOK: 1¾ HOURS

2 large white onions, sliced
1 tbsp apple cider vinegar
500ml fresh chicken or vegetable stock
200ml boiling water
4 sprigs of fresh thyme
3 garlic cloves, sliced
sea salt and freshly ground black pepper

1. Preheat the oven to 160°C/140°C fan/gas mark 3.
2. Dry fry the onions over a medium–high heat in a non-stick ovenproof pan with a lid. Cook for 5–7 minutes, stirring continuously, until the onion softens and browns at the edges.
3. Add the vinegar, stock, boiling water, thyme and garlic and stir well, scraping up any sticky onions from the bottom of the pan.
4. Cover with the lid and transfer to the oven for 1½ hours, by which time the onions will be soft and unctuous. Season with salt and pepper.

TIP: Delicious in Phase 2 served with Parmesan crisps (see Pistou Soup on page 174).

CAULIFLOWER & ROASTED GARLIC SOUP

This beautiful white soup tastes decadent and creamy. The mellow roasted garlic and sweet onion work brilliantly with the subtle flavour of cauliflower. This is a pillowy, velvety white soup that I find supremely comforting and surprisingly satisfying. When I reset, I make a big batch in advance and have it regularly during the day. Not only does it stave off hunger, but it feels like a gentle hug.

SERVES: 2–3
PREP: 10 MINUTES
COOK: 45 MINUTES

florets from 1 large cauliflower
1 large white onion, quartered
1 whole head of garlic
500ml fresh chicken or vegetable stock
a generous grating of fresh whole nutmeg (optional)
fresh chives, to serve
sea salt and freshly ground black pepper

1. Preheat the oven to 180°C/160°C fan/gas mark 4.
2. Put the cauliflower florets and onion into a large ovenproof dish and season with salt and pepper. Add a splash of cold water and cover the dish tightly with foil.
3. Use a sharp knife to cut off the pointed end of the garlic head, together with the tips of the cloves. This will allow you to squeeze the flesh from the skins once cooked. Wrap the head of garlic in foil.
4. Roast the vegetables and garlic for 35–40 minutes until very soft.
5. Once cooked, unwrap the garlic and squeeze the flesh out of the papery skin of the cloves into a saucepan.
6. Add the cooked vegetables and the stock to the pan, mix to combine, then purée to a velvety double cream consistency. Add boiling water if necessary to achieve the right consistency.
7. Season with salt and pepper, plus a generous grating of fresh nutmeg.
8. Serve scattered with fresh chives.

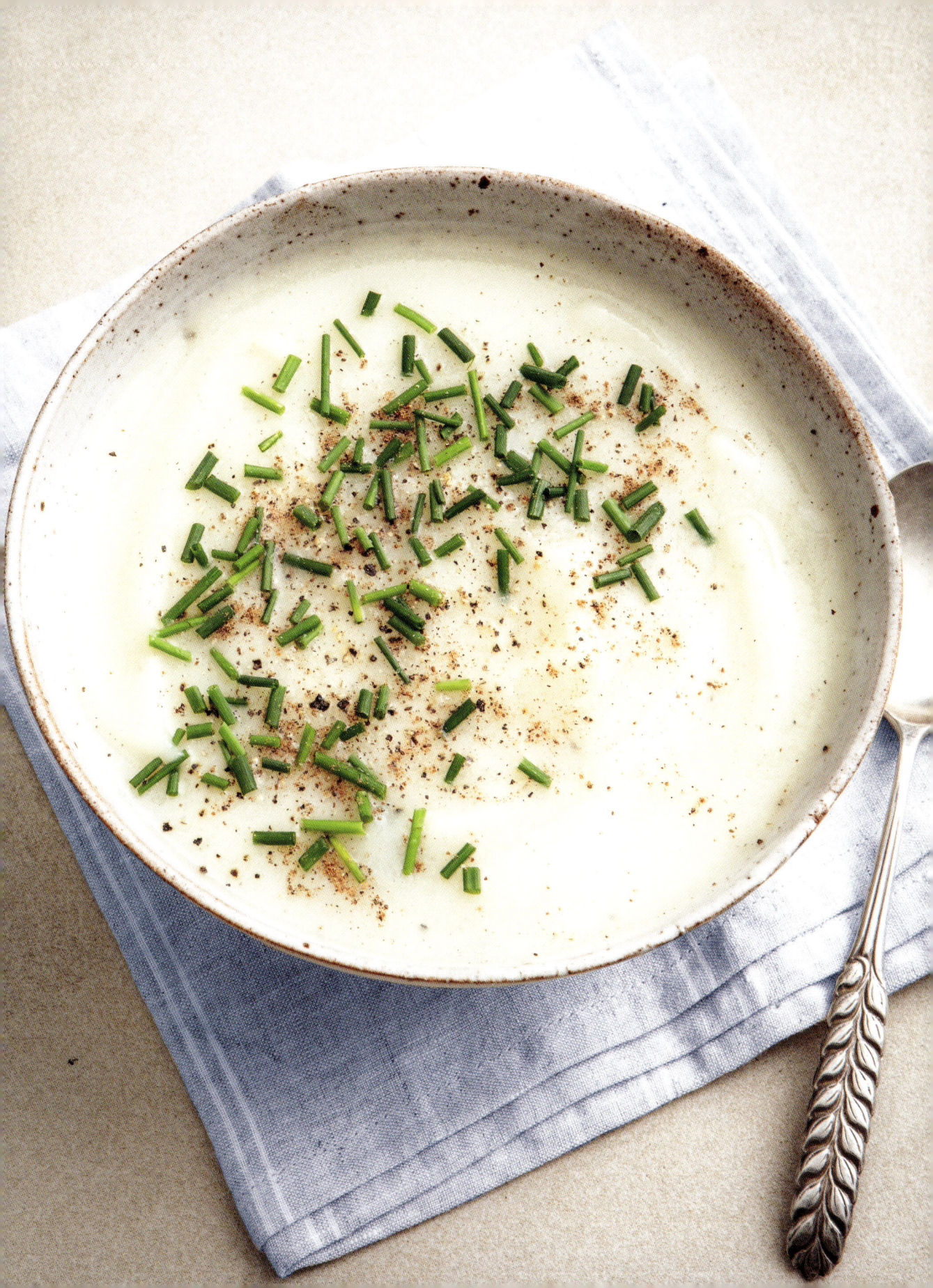

TOMATO CARPACCIO WITH AVOCADO, RED ONION & BASIL

Taking care over the preparation of ingredients can elevate them to something special. Wafer-thin cucumber seasoned with a little sea salt and without its slightly bitter skin is delicate and refreshing. The best tomatoes for this carpaccio have fewer seeds and more flesh, for example bull's eye, beefsteak, rosa or San Marzano. Layer the ingredients and carefully season each layer as you go; the addition of sweet red onion and fresh basil is delicious. This recipe is not suitable for those avoiding nightshades.

SERVES 2
PREP: 15 MINUTES

1 small cucumber, peeled and very thinly sliced
2–3 medium–large tomatoes*, very thinly sliced
2–3 tbsp fresh basil, torn
1 ripe avocado, cubed
¼ red onion, very thinly sliced
2 tsp Pistou (see page 58; optional)
sea salt and freshly ground black pepper

1. Spread the cucumber in a single layer on a large plate and season with a little salt.
2. Layer the thinly-sliced tomatoes on top of the cucumber and season with salt and black pepper.
3. Scatter the torn basil, avocado and red onion on top of the tomatoes and use a teaspoon to dot small amounts of the pistou all over the carpaccio.

TIP: *Put the avocado stone in the middle of the carpaccio and cover the dish tightly to slow down oxidation, so the avocado won't discolour as rapidly.*

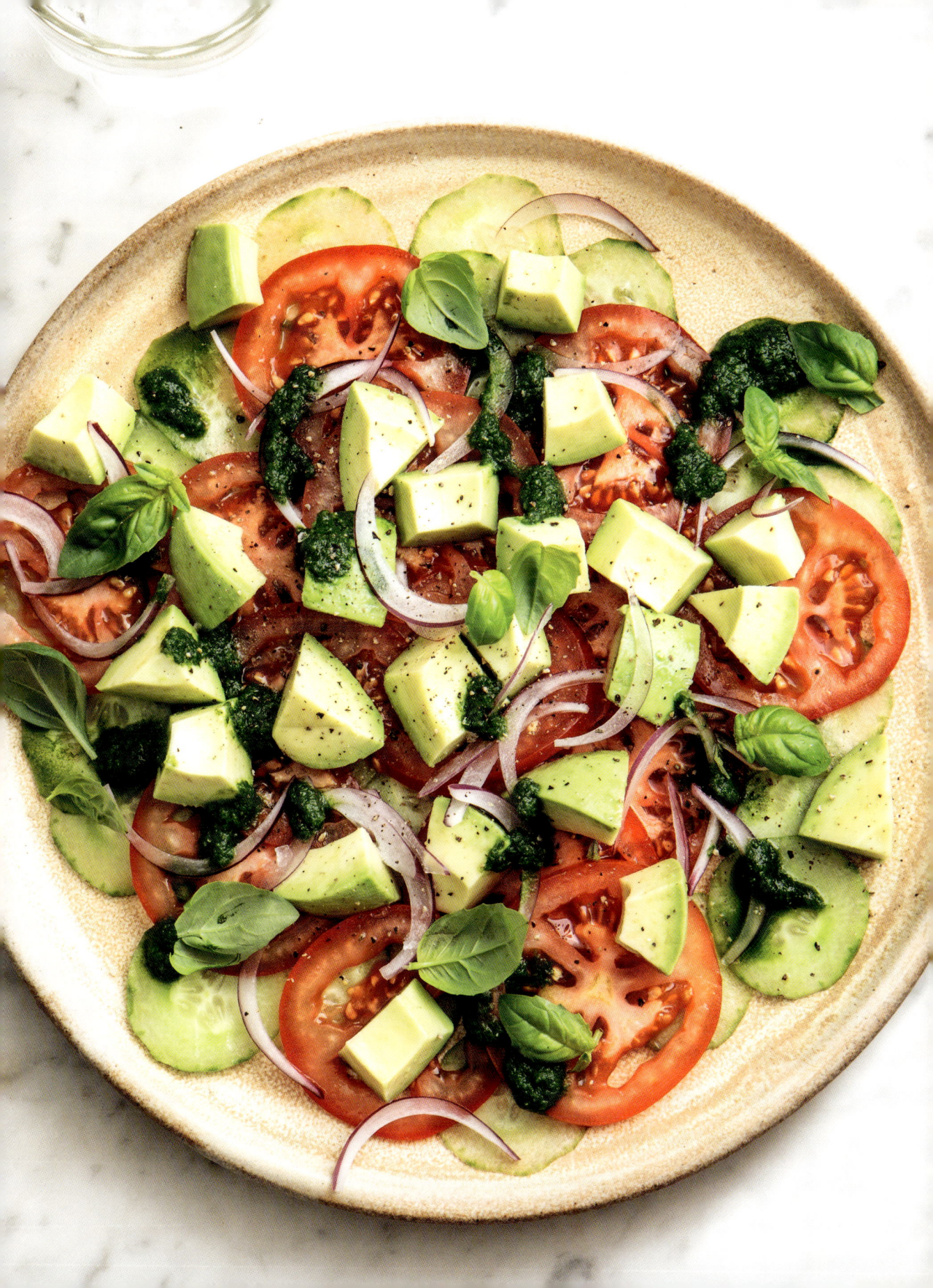

SUNSHINE SAFFRON CAULIFLOWER RICE PILAF

Getting creative with vegetables, spices and herbs is what Phase 1 is all about. This is a quick and easy spin on a pilaf using cauliflower rice, golden veggies and sublimely fragrant saffron. This is great to have ready so you can pop a bowl into the microwave whenever you feel hungry. Serve with a flourish of bright freshly chopped parsley and plenty of black pepper.

SERVES 2
PREP: 10 MINUTES
COOK: 15 MINUTES

40g onion, finely diced
150ml fresh chicken or vegetable stock
70g butternut squash, peeled and finely diced
30g carrot, finely diced
2 sticks of celery, finely diced
2 large garlic cloves, crushed
1 bay leaf
100g cauliflower rice (see page 140)
½ tsp saffron strands, soaked in water for 10 minutes
fresh parsley, chopped, to serve
sea salt and freshly ground black pepper

1. In a non-stick pan with a lid cook the onion in a splash of stock for 4–5 minutes until soft.
2. Add the squash, carrot, celery, garlic, bay leaf and the remaining stock. Cover with a lid and gently simmer for about 6–7 minutes until the veggies soften.
3. Add the cauliflower rice and saffron infused water and continue to cook with the lid off until all the liquid has evaporated – about 5 minutes. Season generously with salt and pepper.
4. Serve with a scattering of fresh parsley.

TIP: Feel free to experiment with any vegetables from the list (see page 68) that you fancy. Chop all vegetables to a similar size to ensure even cooking.

BUTTERNUT SQUASH & GREEN BEAN CURRY

A fresh, light and fragrant curry, mild and gently spiced. Using some of the butternut squash and spiced stock to make the sauce creates substance and pulls the dish together. This curry freezes well.

SERVES
PREP: 10 MINUTES
COOK: 25 MINUTES

½ medium onion, finely diced
2 garlic cloves, finely sliced
2 tsp mild curry powder
1 tsp ground coriander
¼ tsp ground turmeric
300g butternut squash, peeled, deseeded and roughly chopped
250ml fresh chicken or vegetable stock
150g green beans, halved
3 fresh tomatoes*, roughly chopped
fresh coriander, to serve
sea salt and freshly ground black pepper

1. In a non-stick pan, cook the onion in a splash of cold water over a medium heat for about 5 minutes until soft.
2. Add the garlic, spices, butternut squash, stock and a generous pinch of salt. Cover with a lid and simmer over a low heat for 15 minutes.
3. Add the green beans and tomatoes and cook for a further 5 minutes until the butternut squash is tender.
4. Carefully remove 2–3 tablespoons of the squash with a little cooking liquid, and purée until smooth. Pour the purée back into the pan.
5. Check the seasoning, adding more salt and pepper if necessary. Serve with a scattering of coriander.

VARIATION
- You can replace the tomatoes with fresh spinach if you are avoiding nightshades.

RAINBOW SLAW WITH CREAMY AVOCADO DRESSING

This slaw is more than just a pretty face! The delicious combination of red cabbage, carrot, fennel, red onion and fresh herbs doused in apple cider vinegar is jam-packed with powerful antioxidants. Your gut microbiome is going to thank you! The creamy dressing feels indulgent and packs a gentle garlicky and peppery punch. You can use a sharp knife, mandolin or potato peeler to shred the veggies.

SERVES 2–3
PREP: 20 MINUTES

FOR THE SLAW
2 carrots, grated
½ small red cabbage, finely sliced, core removed
1 fennel bulb, finely sliced
¼ red onion, finely sliced
a large handful of herbs, roughly chopped (e.g. chives, dill, parsley, coriander, mint)
1 tbsp apple cider vinegar
generous pinch of sea salt

FOR THE CREAMY AVOCADO DRESSING
½ large ripe avocado
2 tsp apple cider vinegar
½ tsp mustard powder
1 small garlic clove, crushed
splash of cold water
sea salt and freshly ground black pepper

1. To make the rainbow slaw, mix the carrot, cabbage, fennel, onion and herbs in a large bowl. Sprinkle with the vinegar and a generous pinch of sea salt and mix well.
2. For the avocado dressing, blitz all the ingredients, adding small splashes of cold water until you have the consistency you desire.

TIP: *Both the slaw and the dressing are great for all phases. For Phase 2 and beyond, weigh the portion of slaw according to your vegetable allowance. For the dressing in Phase 2, deduct the avocado from your vegetable allowance.*

VARIATION
- If you are not a fan of fennel, you can replace it with white cabbage.

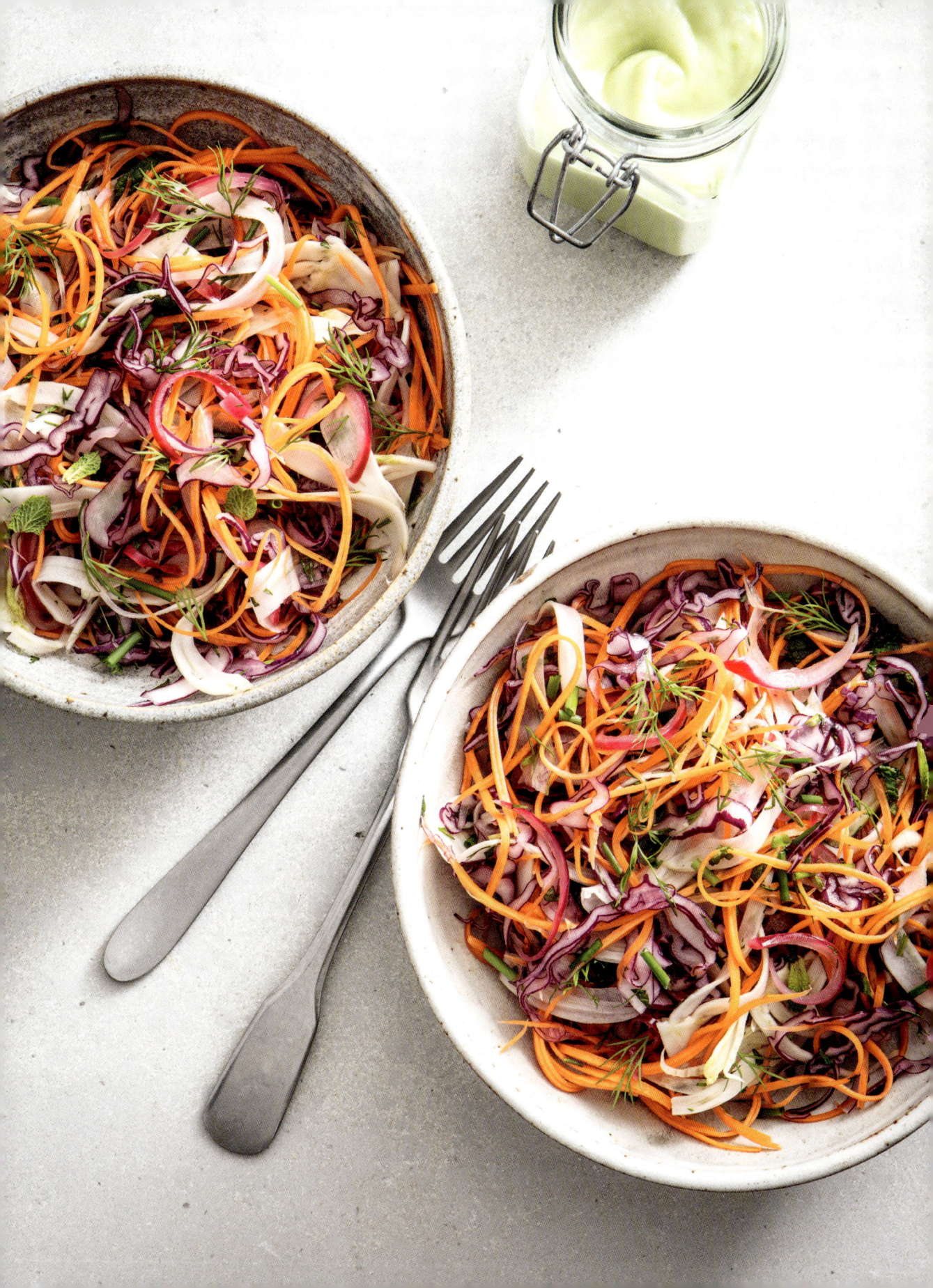

GARLIC BRAISED HISPI CABBAGE WITH CARAMELISED ONIONS

Hispi cabbage is one of my all-time favourite side dishes; it is also the perfect meal during Phase 1 as it feels substantial. The sweetly caramelised onions, fragrant garlic and deep umami flavours of the cabbage are a truly harmonious combination. This is gorgeous as a side dish at any time during Reset.

SERVES 2
PREP: 5 MINUTES
COOK: 45 MINUTES

1 large onion, sliced into wedges
1 pointed cabbage, cut into wedges lengthways
4 garlic cloves, thinly sliced
2 bay leaves
3 sprigs of fresh thyme
300ml fresh chicken or vegetable stock
sea salt and freshly ground black pepper

1. Preheat the oven to 180°C/160°C fan/gas mark 4.
2. Nestle the onion, cabbage, garlic, bay leaves and thyme in a shallow ovenproof dish.
3. Add the stock and season generously with salt and pepper.
4. Bake for 15–20 minutes.
5. When the cabbage begins to char and colour, carefully turn the wedges over and return to the oven. Bake for a further 25–35 minutes until the cabbage is tender, most of the stock has evaporated and the onions are sweetly caramelised.

TIP: When preparing the cabbage include some of the stalk as that will hold the wedges together during cooking.

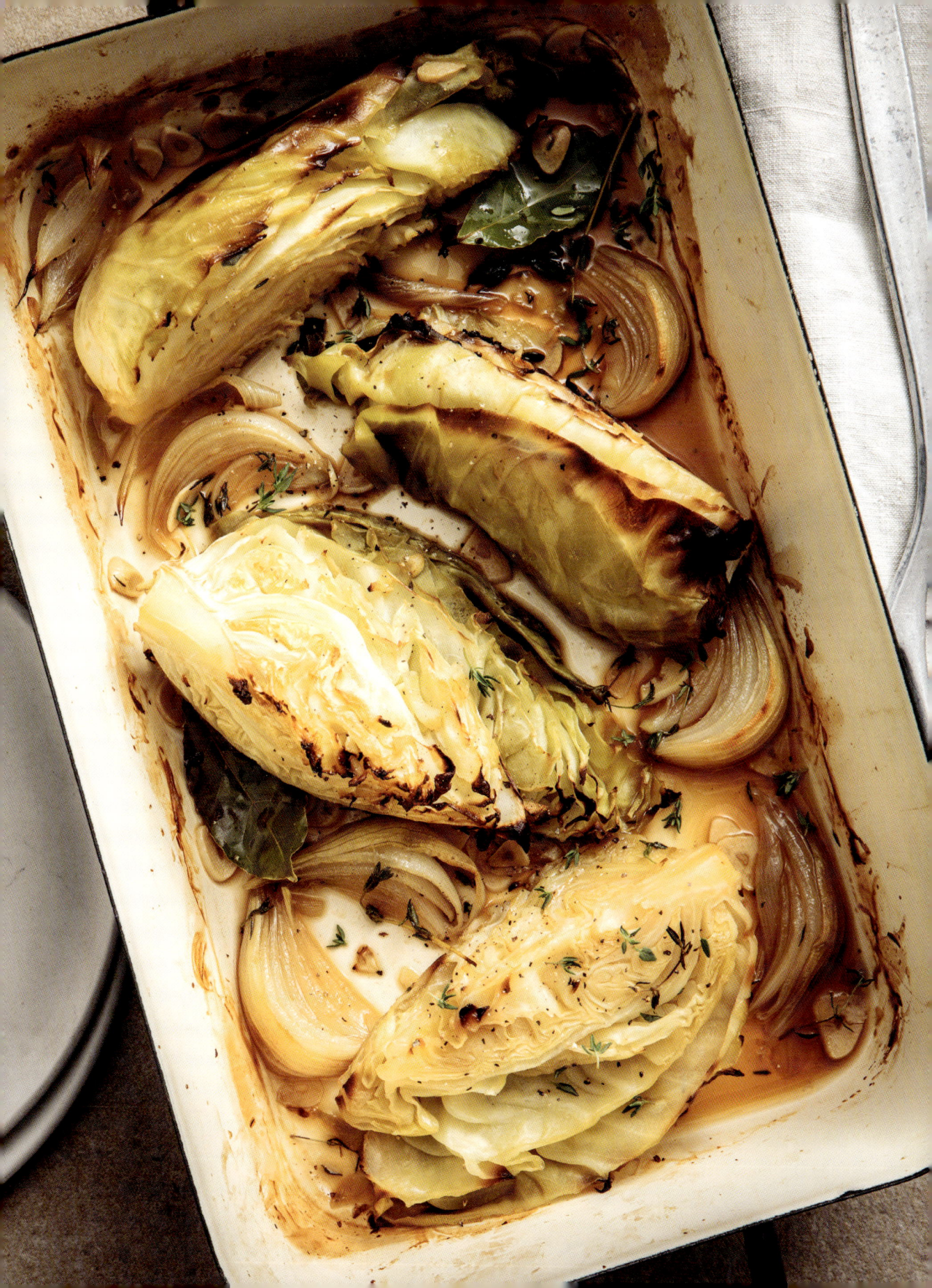

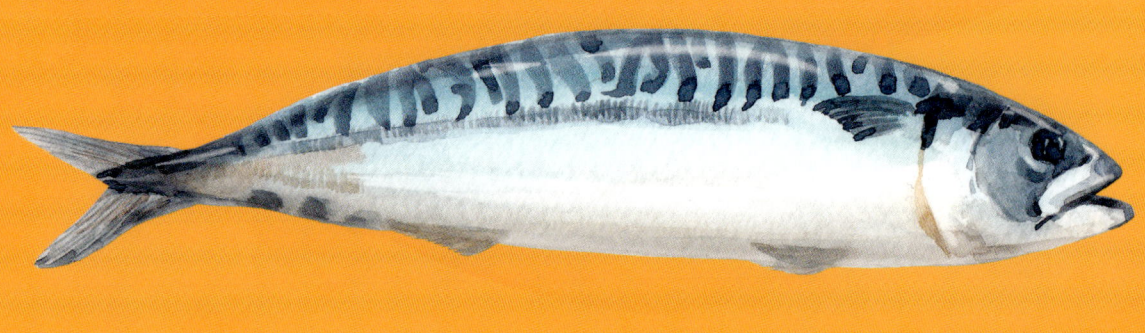
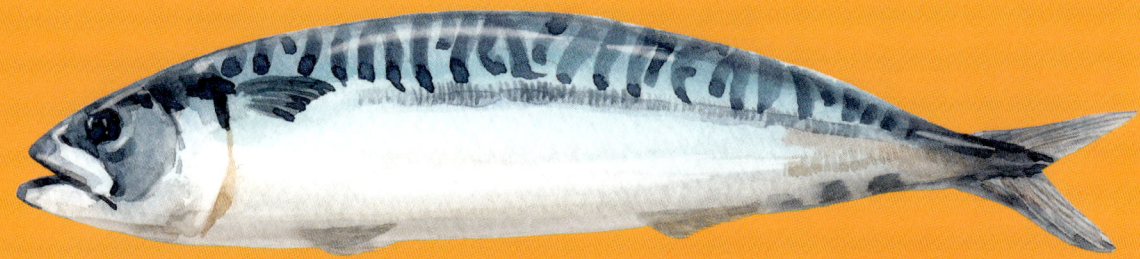
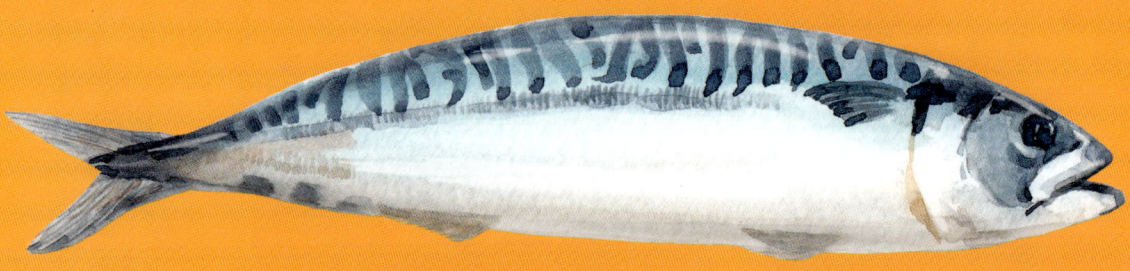
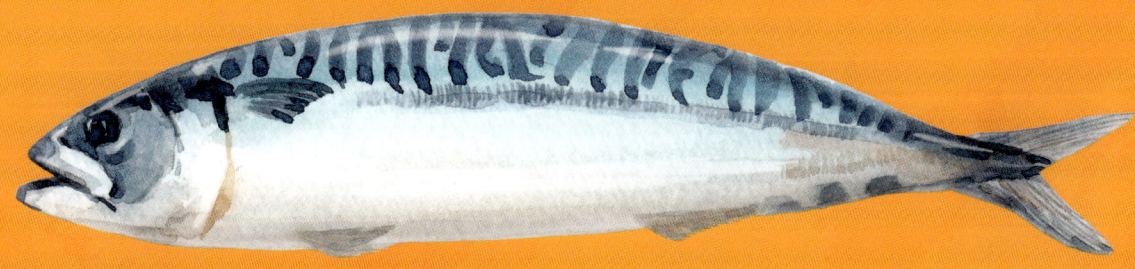

PHASE 2

We're ready to roll!

WELCOME TO PHASE 2

Phase 2 follows the two Phase 1 vegetable days. It begins on day three and is 14 days of sticking like a limpet to the rules below. As for Phase 1, remember that if a food is not listed it's not allowed – if you're wondering whether a food you're hankering after is allowed, check the Phase 2 food list here. The foods included on the list have been tried and tested (in clinical practice and by thousands of HBD followers) and they deliver the biggest nutritional bang for your buck. Stick with these foods and follow the rules and you will get the dazzling results you deserve.

From the first day of Phase 2 onwards you eat three meals a day and fast for five hours between meals – drinking only water between meals and black coffee or tea only with meals. Following two days of vegetables you'll find that eating protein food (eggs, fish, tofu, meat) feels like a luxury; it tastes so good! You are still grain-free, oil-free, alcohol-free and sugar-free (and ideally dairy-free too – see Potentially problematic foods pages 32–33) for another 14 days.

During Reset you're communicating metabolically with your body and changing it from a sugar-burner into a fat-burner so your energy can dip during the first few days of Phase 2. Why is this? It's both because you're detoxing and because your body is no longer getting the carbs and sugar it may have come to rely on. Your brain is messaging: 'Give me food; I've got no fuel here.' And you're replying: 'We're going to be burning fat for energy now – no more sugar!'

But we do make the switch from sugar burning to fat burning and, when we do, it's almost palpable. With that switch your energy returns – you're not just back to normal, you'll find that you have more energy than you have had for ages. Occasionally – thankfully rarely – it takes longer than two weeks for energy to improve. Happily most HBDers tell us that they find their energy level is hugely improved by the end of the Reset.

LIZZIE'S HBD TIPS

Before you know it, you will have reached Phase 2 and the reintroduction of protein will feel like an enormous treat. The first bite of protein in Phase 2 is sensational. Many people choose simple boiled or poached eggs with a few flakes of sea salt along with their vegetables – perhaps as dippy vegetable soldiers on the side. The simplicity of this breakfast is perfection after two days of veggies only.

You may already be noticing that your palate is changing. Eradicating processed foods, condiments and seasonings allows the true flavours of each ingredient to burst into technicolour. Embarking on HBD is a journey of culinary rediscovery. Your daily apple will taste like the nectar of the gods, especially when it's fridge cold and sliced wafer thin.

Petronella advises choosing the highest quality proteins where possible, as she writes in her book (page 85–87 of the second edition). Choose chicken, fish, tofu, eggs and walnuts or seeds over dairy or pulses whenever possible. You may be horrified at the thought of eating meat and fish for breakfast – but a breakfast buffet table in a good hotel nearly always has a meat and smoked fish section.

Meat: I wouldn't suggest beef stew for breakfast; however, a cold chicken salad with leaves, cucumber, fresh herbs and slivers of fridge cold grapes is a thing of joy.

Fish: smoked mackerel and smoked salmon are both breakfast staples on the continent. Serve simply with 80g avocado and make up the right veggie weight with mixed salad leaves and a squeeze of lemon. Smoked haddock or kippers grilled and served with snipped chives are delicious with a salad of leaves, simply tossed in apple cider vinegar and sea salt.

Eggs: boiled, scrambled or fried, eggs are a mainstay HBD breakfast for many. Rustle up a quick omelette stuffed with mushrooms, courgettes and fresh herbs. Alternatively baked eggs are another great oil free dish in Phase 2. The Baked Green Eggs recipe on page 129 is undoubtedly my favourite and ideal for batch cooking; useful for busy mornings when you're short of time.

Walnuts and seeds: walnuts become slightly crisp when briefly toasted in a dry pan; they make a brilliant quick breakfast with fresh raspberries and a black coffee laced with cinnamon. Chopped toasted walnuts create a delicious topping for warm baked cherries or spiced apples. Another much-loved HBD classic breakfast is a grated apple with cinnamon and ground or whole toasted pumpkin and sunflower seeds.

Dairy: if you're eating yoghurt, remember, whether it's from a sheep, goat or cow, it should always be full-fat Greek style. Serve with berries or frozen cherries warmed briefly in the microwave or in a pan on the hob, and sprinkled with cinnamon and vanilla. A wedge of sharp, salty Cheddar, some crudites and an apple for breakfast is great when you're in a hurry, along with a cup of green tea.

Coffee: if you are a coffee lover like me, I promise that you will quickly adjust to having black coffee. I now much prefer the clean, bitter notes and can't believe I used to drown it in dairy – and way too much sugar. As with everything HBD, black coffee needn't be boring. Add a little cinnamon and nutmeg to a mug of hot coffee for a gentle spicy note, or a pinch of vanilla to sweeten. Alternatively, try an HBD espresso martini: whizz up half a teaspoon of vanilla powder or cinnamon and a shot of black coffee over ice in a blender. The result is almost creamy – an intense and gorgeous alternative on a hot day.

The premise of HBD cookery is choosing the most natural and nutritious ingredients and turning them into meals that satisfy your soul and senses, as well as nuturing your physical well-being. Many of the recipes designed for HBD will become your all-time favourite dishes, meals that you will gladly choose to eat time and again.

PHASE 2 RULES

- Eat three meals a day and fast for at least five hours between each meal – water only during the five hours
- Begin each meal with a bite of protein and only eat one type of protein per meal
- All foods are weighed before cooking – for most people, this is usually 100g of vegetables and 100g of protein for breakfast, and 130g of vegetables and 130g of protein for main meals, but see the note on page 104 and the Breakfast and Main Meal Planners on pages 102–103 for more details
- No added oil and no alcohol
- No wheat or any other grains
- No cardio or intense exercise – see below
- Drink the right amount of water (35ml per kilo of body weight)
- Eat one apple, with or after a meal, once a day
- Don't eat for longer than one hour (coffee or tea count as part of your meal)
- Finish eating by 9pm (and the earlier the better)
- No sugar (and no honey, stevia or fake sugar)

One surefire way to sabotage your efforts with HBD is to overdo exercise. Intense exercise is a stressor and increases cortisol, which not only makes fat burning difficult – it also increases inflammation and puts us into fight or flight mode. What you're aiming for in the all important Reset is to spend more time in the parasympathetic nervous system – this is the place for resting, digesting and repairing. You will naturally find that you have temporarily lower energy levels in Phase 2 while your body is searching for fuel and before it becomes good at burning fat for energy. Also intense exercise can make us hungrier – so it's walking all the way. Stretching, gentle yoga, Tai chi and Pilates are all also perfect.

Note: To understand the reasoning and rationale behind the rules, read the bible, *The Human Being Diet* and read it again. The better you understand the reasoning, the easier it is to stay on track and to give the programme your all. Really understanding HBD is key to ensuring your success and astounding results.

PHASE 2 FOOD LIST – IF IT'S NOT LISTED IT'S NOT ALLOWED!

Weigh all food before cooking

Note: yoghurt and cheese are included here only for those who've eliminated dairy in the past and know they're OK with it.

Protein foods	One type of protein per meal
Fish (fresh or smoked)	All including cod, kippers, haddock, halibut, mackerel, plaice, red mullet, salmon, sardines (fresh), sea bass, sea bream, skate, snapper, sole, tilapia, trout, tuna (canned in water or fresh), turbot
Poultry (breast meat only, no skin)	chicken, turkey, pheasant or lean duck breast
Seafood	clams, crab, lobster, mussels, oysters, prawns, scallops, squid
Red meat (remove visible fat) – no gammon, bacon, sausages, ham or dried meats	Twice a week max – unprocessed and fresh beef, lamb, pork or venison (and any fresh, lean wild or game meat). Grass-fed and organic when possible.
Pulses	lentils, chickpeas, cannellini/butter beans/haricot beans – avoid edamame beans. All pulses (unless bought cooked or canned) must be well cooked.
Soy	tofu, tempeh or natto (fermented soy protein)
Seeds (breakfast only)	sunflower and pumpkin seeds, ground or whole
Nuts (breakfast only)	walnuts
Eggs	Up to 14 per week (you can have two eggs for lunch or dinner as long as you haven't had them for breakfast).
Yoghurt (breakfast only)	Full-fat unsweetened unflavoured, sheep, cow or goat. Or soy yoghurt for vegans only. Ensure that dairy yoghurt is minimum 9g (9%) protein and 5g fat (5%) per 100g and maximum 4g (4%) carbs
Cheese (cow, goat or sheep – no soy or nut cheese)	Traditional cheeses, including brie, Cheddar, Edam, feta, gorgonzola, Gouda, gruyere, halloumi, manchego, mozzarella, Parmesan, stilton (no ultra-processed cheeses)

Aim for 3 different vegetables with each meal

Vegetables	
Note the max weights of avocado and tomatoes Olives should be pitted and included within your vegetable weight *denotes nightshade	artichokes (fresh or bottled in brine), asparagus, aubergines*, avocado (max 80g per meal), broccoli, Brussels sprouts, butternut squash (and all other types of squash), cabbages, capers (in brine, sugar-free), carrots, cauliflower, celery, chicory, Chinese leaf lettuce, courgettes, cress, cucumbers, endive, fennel, fresh herbs (all), gherkins or dill pickles (sugar-free), green beans, kale, kimchi*, kohlrabi, leeks, lettuce (all including iceberg, romaine, lamb's lettuce), mushrooms, okra, olives (max 4 in a meal), onions, pak choi, peppers*, radishes, rocket, romanesco, samphire, sauerkraut, seaweed, shallots, spring greens, spring onions, spinach, tomatoes* (max 30g per day)

One type of fruit per meal from this list as an option – no mixing and no other types of fruit

Fruit	
1 apple with one meal once a day Lemon can be squeezed over fish or chicken, as long as there's no other fruit in that meal	apples (x1), blueberries, blackberries, cherries, grapes, mangoes, papayas, plums, pomegranate seeds, raspberries, strawberries (maximum 100g per meal) Fruit, other than a daily apple, is included as an optional extra; it doesn't replace the protein or veg in your meal

Phase 2 optional extras	
Black coffee, black/green/white/rooibos tea, herbal tea (no fruit tea) with meals only	No added milk of any kind, sugar or sweeteners
Seasoning	Fresh, dried, frozen herbs and spices e.g. chilli*, ginger, garlic, turmeric, sea salt, Himalayan salt, pepper, mustard powder, fresh horseradish HBD purists avoid tamari (gluten-free soy sauce) until Phase 3 to allow their tastebuds to revive
Apple cider vinegar – unpasteurised, organic and with 'the mother' with meals only	Add to food or mix into water for a refreshing drink
Clear chicken or vegetable stock	Liquid only, no stock cubes/bouillon powder – see pages 62–63 for homemade stock recipes

Smoked fish weights are for fresh fish with the exception of smoked salmon (sugar-free of course). Eat 75g for breakfast, with 100g vegetables, or 100g for main meals with 130g vegetables.

> *Nightshade vegetables are marked with an asterisk. Recipes that include nightshade vegetables are marked with 🌶.

AN EXAMPLE OF A PERFECT HBD PHASE 2 DAY

7am: hop out of bed and drink at least half a litre of water. Then shower, dress and get ready for your day.

8am at the latest: aim to eat within an hour of waking. Breakfast followed by (optional) black tea or coffee. Breakfast might be two eggs with spinach, avocado and mushrooms, or 35g walnuts with a grated apple – see the food list, recipes and meal planners for ideas.

Drink lots of water between breakfast and lunch and fast for at least five hours from the end of breakfast to the beginning of lunch.

12.30/12.45pm: walk for at least 10 minutes before lunch.

1–1.30pm: lunch followed by (optional) black tea or coffee. Lunch might be 130g salmon or tofu with 130g mixed leaves, fennel and avocado. Or Houmous with Crudités (see page 205). Apple cider vinegar can be added to your food or water. Remember to start counting your five hour fast from the last bite of food and the last sip of tea or coffee.

Drink water only between lunch and dinner and fast for at least five hours from the end of lunch to the beginning of dinner.

6.30/6.45pm: another walk, 10 minutes minimum, before dinner.

7–7.30pm: dinner followed by (optional) herbal tea. Dinner might be prawns with salad and vegetables or Shiitake Mushroom, Spinach & Thyme Risotto (see page 142).

10pm: bed!

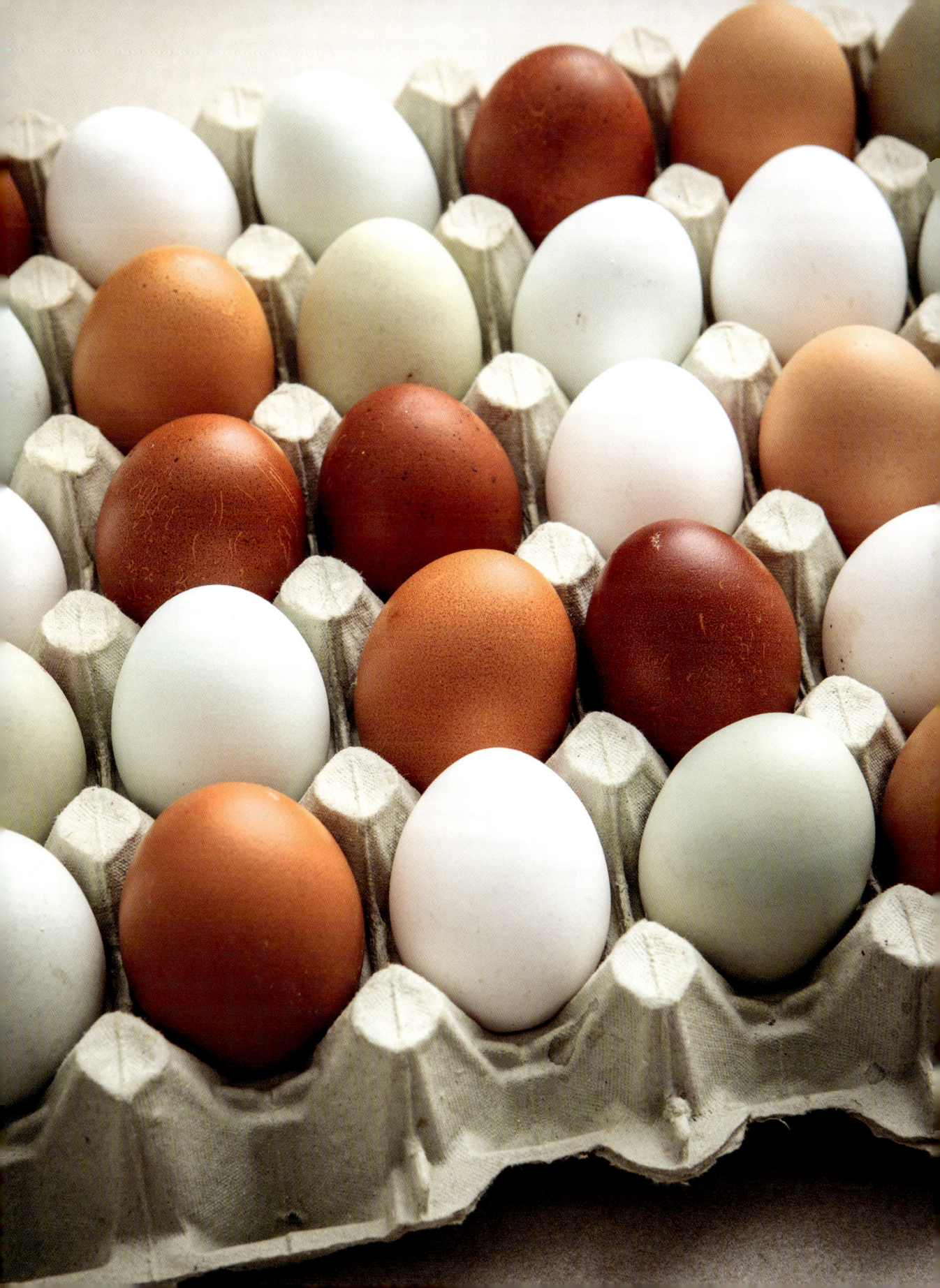

BREAKFAST PLANNER

Note: yoghurt and cheese are only included below for experienced HBDers who know that these foods suit them.

Breakfast 1
2 eggs
100g vegetables

Breakfast 2
35g sunflower and pumpkin seeds or 35g walnuts
1 apple or 100g fruit and/or 100g veg

Breakfast 3
100g chicken or turkey breast (no skin)
100g vegetables

Breakfast 4
75g smoked salmon or 100g fresh fish
100g vegetables

Breakfast 5
100g tofu or tempeh
100g vegetables

Breakfast 6
100g fresh salmon (or other fish)
100g vegetables

Breakfast 7
120g pulses (cooked or canned weight) or 60g dried weight
100g vegetables

Breakfast 8
160g full fat yoghurt
100g fruit and/or 100g veg

Breakfast 9
60g cheese
100g vegetables

MAIN MEAL PLANNER

Note: cheese is only included below for experienced HBDers who know that it suits them.

Lunch/Dinner 1
130g tofu or tempeh
130g vegetables

Lunch/Dinner 2
130g fish or seafood (or 100g smoked salmon)
130g vegetables

Lunch/Dinner 3
130g turkey or chicken breast (no skin)
130g vegetables

Lunch/Dinner 4
130g meat (red meat x2/week max)
130g vegetables

Lunch/Dinner 5
160g pulses (cooked or canned weight) or 80g dried weight
130g vegetables

Lunch/Dinner 6
2 eggs (but not if you had them for breakfast!)
130g vegetables

Lunch/Dinner 7
80g cheese (but not if you had yoghurt for breakfast)
130g vegetables

A note on food weights

If you weigh less than 65kg you can take 10g off the protein and vegetable weights, for example, have 120g meat and 120g vegetables or 70g cheese with 120g vegetables. If you weigh more than 80kg you can add 10g to the weights above, for example, have 140g meat and 140g vegetables, or 90g cheese with 140g vegetables.

Breakfast weights remain the same for everyone. Smoked fish weights are the same as fresh fish with the exception of smoked salmon (sugar-free of course). Eat 75g for breakfast, with 100g vegetables, or 100g for main meals with 130g vegetables.

No substitutions!

One of the questions we are often asked is: 'can I have almond or oat milk in my tea or coffee?' Or: 'can I have dairy milk in my coffee if I'm having yoghurt for breakfast?' And the answer is always no! You need to get used to drinking it black. If you can't bear black coffee opt for green tea instead. Otherwise once you're in Phase 4 and out for coffee with friends you'll be breaking your fast with a milky tea or coffee – it's essentially a mini meal containing natural sugars and fats. Fasting between meals is one of the HBD cardinal rules.

> Don't allow yourself to be derailed – crashing out of Phase 2 means starting again and you definitely don't want to do that – give it your all.

LIZZIE'S HBD TIPS

HBD RICE & PASTA
HBD rice and HBD pasta (e.g. Biona or Mr Organic) is made with 100% lentil or chickpea flour, which is the protein part of your meal. The rice tastes a little like orzo pasta. It has a lovely bite and makes a fabulous, fuss free risotto, as unlike standard rice, there is no need for constant stirring. To make a basic risotto with chickpea rice, cook onions and garlic in a splash of stock, add the rice and more stock and simmer for about 20 minutes until the rice is al dente and all the liquid has evaporated. Play around with the flavours and add the vegetables and herbs and spices of your choice.

Another easy store cupboard staple, chickpea pasta is so versatile. Cook and serve tossed in Red Pepper Ketchup (see page 56), as long as you're not avoiding nightshades, as well as torn basil leaves and roasted tenderstem broccoli. Alternatively, simmer sofrito (diced onion, celery and carrot) in chicken stock until the vegetables are tender and the stock is reduced. Add cooked pasta, fresh herbs, a good squeeze of lemon and season well.

STEWS & CASSEROLES
Stews and casseroles are especially useful in Phase 2 as they can be made without oil. They are perfect for batch cooking at the weekend to freeze for the week ahead. However, one of the challenges can be how to thicken a stew without flour: is a stew even a stew without a proper sauce?

Reducing method
Once your stew is cooked, remove the meat and vegetables and keep them warm. Briskly boil the residual cooking liquid to reduce it until it darkens in colour and thickens to become syrupy. This will create an intensely flavoured sauce to pour back over the meat and veggies.

Puréeing
This is how to add a velvety texture when making bean stews and casseroles. When making a bean stew, remove a spoonful of the beans with a little cooking liquid and puree it until smooth. Pour it back into your stew, creating a silky sauce. You can do the same with softly cooked butternut squash in a chicken stew or fish curry.

Bread

Eliminating wheat can feel like a huge step when you first embark on your HBD journey. Indeed, along with a chilled Provence rose, I missed bread the most when I first embarked on HBD!

However, I then discovered socca breads. These are flatbreads made from chickpea flour (also known as gram flour) and they have a distinct nutty flavour and are brilliant dunked into vegetable stews or soups. Crucially, they really hit the spot when you are craving something filling.

To make a simple socca bread whisk 80g of chickpea flour with 130ml of cold water, and salt and pepper to create a batter with the consistency of double cream. Heat a non-stick frying pan and drop a tablespoon of batter at a time on to the hot pan. After 2 minutes little bubbles will appear on the surface of the bread. Flip and cook the other side for 1–2 minutes; repeat until you have 8–10 small flatbreads; there is no need for oil.

KINDNESS

Just as important as nurturing yourself with delicious and comforting food is to be kind and gentle to yourself during Reset. Focusing on what brings you joy and helps you to relax will support the transformation that is happening in your body. Comfort can be a long bath, a good book, a new box set on Netflix or a gentle stroll in the sunshine.

TREATS

There are often more treats around when everyone is at home. To help you stay on track, plan a few HBD treats just for you. Add a splash or a tablespoon of apple cider vinegar to icy cold sparking water in a wine glass to accompany meals – HBD champagne! Not only is apple cider vinegar proven to counter wine and sugar cravings, it's also great for digestion and makes a delicious and refreshing change from plain water.

I always have a stash of frozen grapes in the freezer. The freezing process transforms grapes into little baubles of sweet sorbet, which are a deliciously simple pudding. Perfect for when everyone else is tucking into ice cream and pudding after supper so you don't feel left out.

YOUR WHYS?

Remember that there's magic in these 14 days of Phase 2, and the Reset must be treated as sacrosanct and completed without interruption. Your brain and body will be ever grateful to you for successfully completing these vitally important two weeks before you head into Phase 3. This is the beginning of your metabolic reset and a whole new vibrantly healthy experience of life. If you find yourself feeling a bit wobbly always bring your attention back to your WHYs and you are set for success:

What are my WHYs? What are my goals? What do I want to change about how I feel? Why is making these changes important to me? How will changing how I feel change my life?

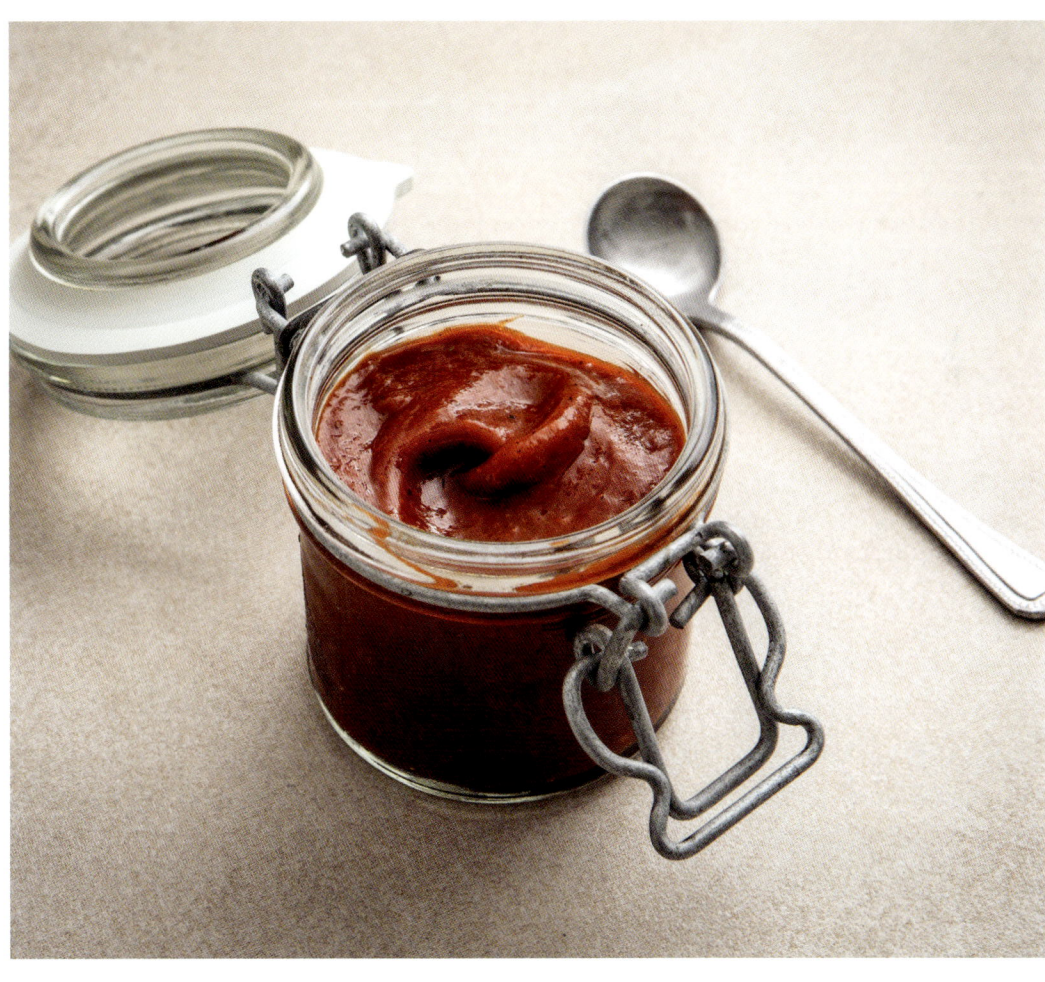

PHASE 2

Breakfasts

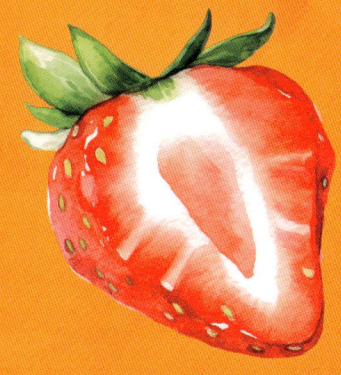

BREAKFAST SLAW

On weekday mornings when you're in a hurry, it's useful to have some delicious breakfasts prepped in the fridge. Make a batch of basic slaw from grated carrot, shredded red and white cabbage and a little onion and ring the changes with different additions each morning. Here I've added toasted walnuts and apple, but it's also delicious with toasted seeds or nuggets of halloumi. Swap the apple for pears or grapes and try adding other soft herbs; parsley and coriander also work well.

SERVES 2
PREP: 10 MINUTES

80g carrots, grated
50g red cabbage, shredded
50g white cabbage, shredded
20g spring onion, finely chopped
2 apples, sliced into small cubes
70g walnuts, lightly toasted
1–2 tbsp fresh chives, finely chopped
sea salt

1. Combine the carrots, red and white cabbage, spring onion and a pinch of sea salt.
2. Add the apple, walnuts and chives and eat immediately.

TIPS: *Use a potato peeler or mandolin to shred the cabbage. Toast the walnuts in a non-stick pan over a medium heat for 3–5 minutes.*

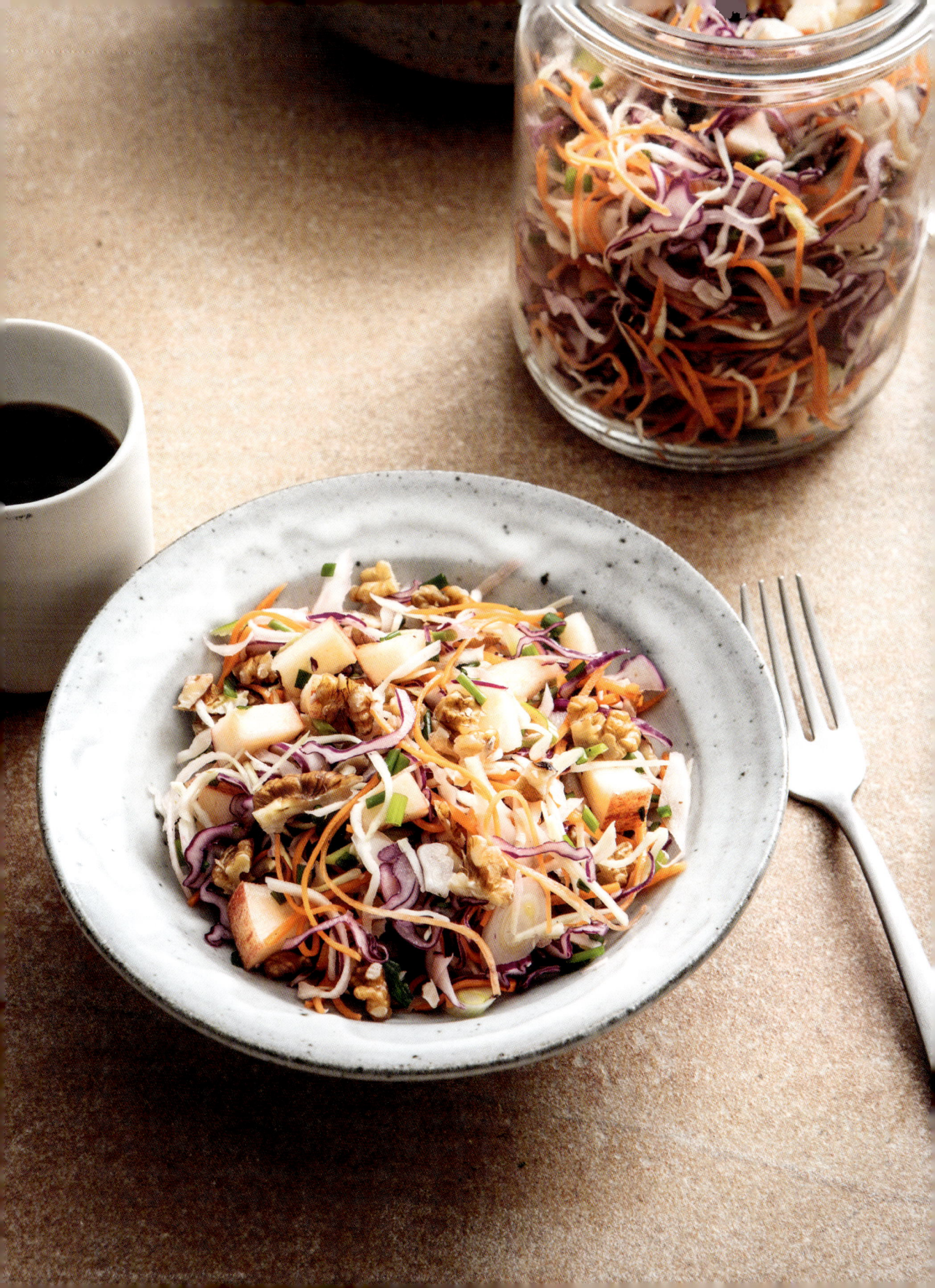

WALDORF SALAD

The original Waldorf salad contained just celery, apple and mayonnaise; the walnuts came later. It has changed a great deal in the 140 years since its inception at the Waldorf Astoria in New York. This Phase 2 variation omits the creamy mayonnaise dressing. I've swapped the crunchy apple for ripe pears, which balance the slightly bitter walnuts and provide moisture in the absence of a dressing. The key is to use ripe fruit, while the celery, cucumber and radish bring crisp freshness.

SERVES 2
PREP: 10 MINUTES

80g celery, thinly sliced
80g radishes, halved and thinly sliced
40g cucumber, thinly sliced
1–2 tbsp finely chopped fresh chives
200g ripe pear, sliced into small cubes
70g walnuts, lightly toasted for 3–5 minutes in a non-stick pan
sea salt

1. Combine the celery, radishes, cucumber and chives and sprinkle with a pinch of salt.
2. Add the pear and walnuts and eat immediately.

TIP: Make a batch of salad to store in the fridge, then add the pears and walnuts fresh each morning. Thinly sliced fridge-cold green grapes can replace the pear.

AVOCADO & SMOKED SALMON SALAD

A speedy yet decadent breakfast that bursts with flavours and textures. Chopping the salad leaves and vegetables small ensures that you have a combination of flavours in every forkful. Peppery rocket, sweet red onion, cool cucumber and the earthy notes of parsley and chives balance the rich, oily fish and creamy avocado. Capers, with their unique tangy flavour and firm texture, are delicious with smoked fish. Your gut microbiome will love this too.

SERVES 2
PREP: 5 MINUTES

50g rocket, finely chopped
30g cucumber, peeled and finely chopped
20g red onion, finely chopped
1 tbsp chopped flat-leaf parsley
100g avocado, sliced
150g smoked salmon, sliced
juice of ½ lemon
2–3 tsp capers (sugar-free in brine)
1 tbsp finely chopped fresh chives
freshly ground black pepper

1. Mix the rocket, cucumber, red onion and parsley and pile the mixture on to a serving dish.
2. Top with the sliced avocado and the smoked salmon.
3. Squeeze the lemon juice over the fish and avocado, spoon over the capers, scatter with chives and finish with a generous grind of black pepper.

CUCUMBER, GRAPE & DILL SALAD WITH TZATZIKI

As an alternative to yoghurt and berries, this twist on a savoury Greek classic makes a refreshing and delicious change at breakfast time. The creamy, savoury tzatziki has subtle garlic, cucumber and herb notes, and provides a fabulous contrast to the super sweet and juicy grapes. You can prepare the tzatziki in advance as it keeps well in the fridge for 2–3 days. Stir well before eating.

SERVES 2
PREP: 10 MINUTES

FOR THE TZATZIKI
100g cucumber, deseeded and grated
320g full-fat natural Greek yoghurt
1 small garlic clove, crushed
1–2 tbsp fresh dill, chopped
a pinch of sea salt

FOR THE SALAD
50g cucumber, deseeded and diced
20g spring onion, finely sliced
30g celery, finely sliced
150g fridge cold green grapes, sliced
fresh dill, to serve

1. Make the tzatziki. Use kitchen paper to squeeze as much moisture as possible from the grated cucumber (to prevent the tzatziki becoming watery). Put in a bowl with the yoghurt, garlic, fresh dill and sea salt and mix well.
2. In a separate bowl, combine the salad ingredients.
3. To serve, spoon the tzatziki into a serving dish, pile the salad on top and finish with a scattering of fresh dill and a grind of black pepper.

VARIATION
- Swap the dill for fresh mint.

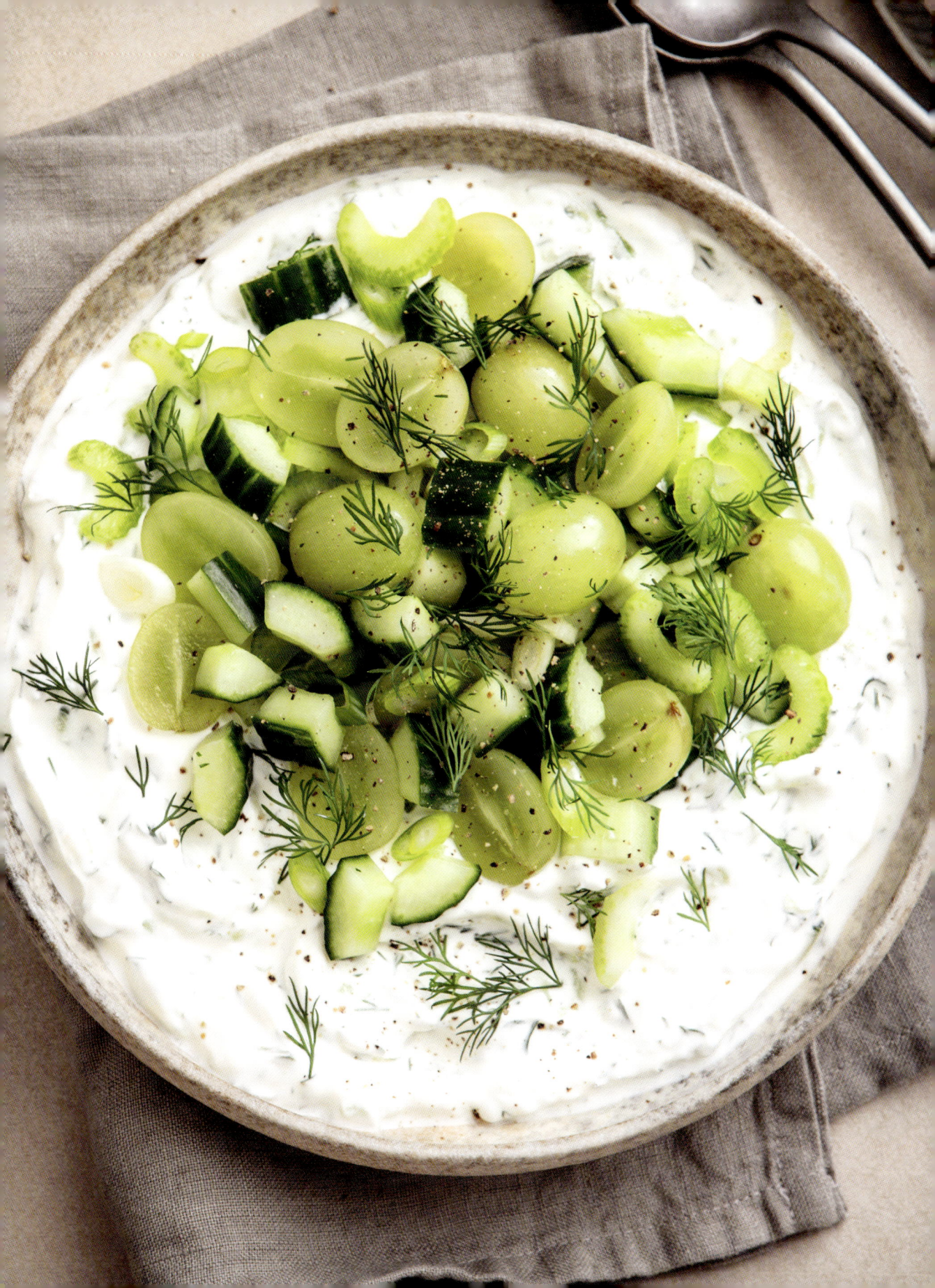

SMOKED MACKEREL SUSHI

Don't be deceived, these gorgeous little sushi rolls may sound complicated to make, but they are incredibly easy. Cucumber ribbons are rolled around smoky fish, heady with the flavours of fresh coriander and lemon. They look glorious and taste even better – and they are an excellent vessel for any combination of fish or seafood. They are delicious with crab and chives or poached salmon and dill.

SERVES 2
PREP: 15 MINUTES

120g cucumber
200g smoked mackerel
zest and juice of 1 lemon
40g spring onion, finely chopped
40g celery, finely chopped
2 tbsp fresh coriander, roughly chopped
freshly ground black pepper

TIP: See Summer Rolls (see page 199) for a photo showing the cucumber wraps.

1. Use a potato peeler to peel down the length of a cucumber and create long even-sized ribbons. Overlap the ribbons on a piece of foil or parchment paper to form a sheet of cucumber to use as the wrapper.
2. Flake the fish into a bowl and add the lemon zest and juice, spring onion, celery, coriander and a generous grind of black pepper. Mix well.
3. Make a sausage shape with the filling across the width of the cucumber wrapper, about a third of the way up. Use the foil or parchment paper to roll it up as firmly as possible, in the same way you would roll a sausage roll.
4. Slice the roll into sections and serve immediately.

VARIATION
- Replace the celery with finely diced radish for a more peppery flavour.

GREEK SALAD

The rich, tangy cheese and briny black olives in this Greek salad negate any need for olive oil. Keep the tomatoes to a minimum; I suggest cutting them into small pieces, guaranteeing a tomatoey morsel in each bite. Peel and deseed the cucumber to stop the salad becoming soggy; this elevates the whole dish. Dried oregano, sea salt and freshly squeezed lemon juice keep the salad vibrant and the flavours authentically Greek. This recipe is not suitable for those avoiding nightshades.

SERVES 2
PREP: 10 MINUTES

80g cucumber, peeled, halved, deseeded and sliced
40g tomato*, chopped into small pieces
60g red pepper*, chopped
20g red onion, finely sliced
8 black olives, halved
120g feta cheese
½ tsp dried oregano
lemon juice
sea salt

1. Combine the cucumber, tomato, red pepper, red onion and olives in a bowl with a pinch of sea salt.
2. Top the salad with the feta, a sprinkle of dried oregano and a squeeze of lemon juice.

TIP: Greek salad also makes a delicious lunch or dinner. Follow the instructions above, adjusting the quantities in line with your own HBD allowance.

HALLOUMI, STRAWBERRY & MINT SALAD

A glorious combination of sweet, juicy strawberries, tangy halloumi and cool mint. Halloumi is great for Phase 2 as it is best dry-fried, without any need for oil. Initially, the liquid from the cheese seeps out during the cooking, but once this evaporates, a delicious golden, chewy crust forms. This little salad is a taste of summer, abundant with herbs and leaves and packed with vitamins, antioxidants and delicious gut-loving fresh herbs.

SERVES 2
PREP: 10 MINUTES
COOK: 5 MINUTES

80g rocket
100g cucumber, peeled and chopped
20g red onion, finely sliced
120g halloumi, cut into 2–3cm slices
100g strawberries, hulled and sliced
3–4 fresh mint leaves, torn

1. Combine the rocket, cucumber and red onion and pile them on to a serving dish.
2. Warm a large non-stick frying pan over a medium heat and add the halloumi. Allow the milky liquid from the cheese to evaporate and turn the slices with a spatula until they are golden on both sides. This will take about 5 minutes. Remove from the heat and allow to cool; the cheese should be warm, not searingly hot.
3. Pile the strawberries on to the rocket and cucumber, then top with the warm cheese and torn mint leaves. Eat immediately.

TIP: *This is also delicious for lunch or dinner; increase quantities in line with your HBD allowance.*

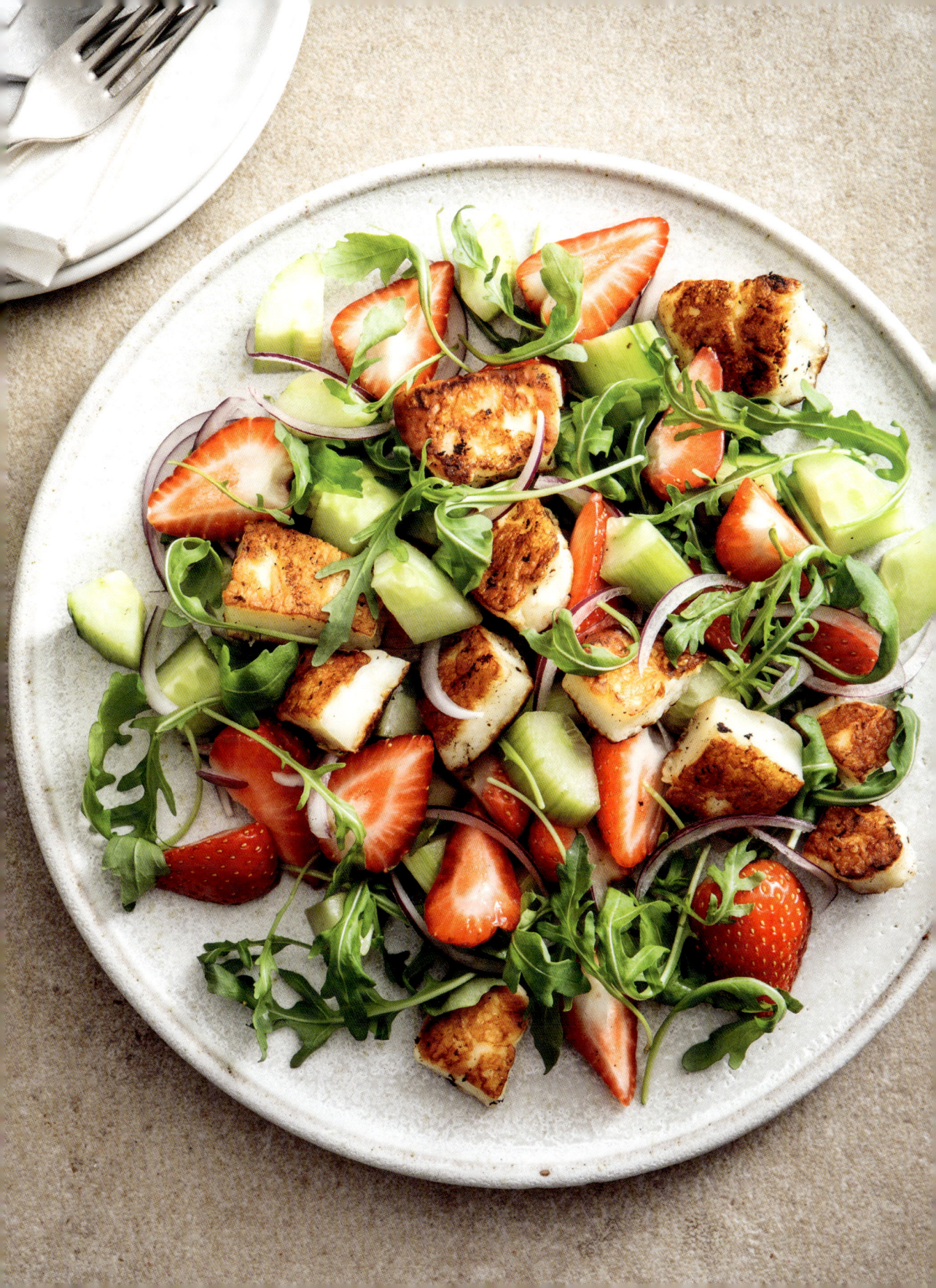

SHREDDED CHICKEN & TARRAGON SALAD

Eating high-quality protein at every meal is proven to keep you fuller for longer and also helps to stabilise blood sugar and boost energy. This recipe was devised on a Monday morning when the fridge contained only leftover chicken from Sunday lunch, some salad and a lone avocado. Blending avocado with fresh tarragon and citrussy lemon creates a creamy dressing that transforms the chicken, while the green salad and extra herbs add freshness and balance.

SERVES 2
PREP: 10 MINUTES

100g avocado
zest and juice of ½ lemon
½ tsp Colman's mustard powder
1 tsp chopped fresh tarragon
200g cooked chicken, shredded
20g rocket
20g spring onion, sliced
20g cucumber, chopped
40g lettuce, shredded
fresh tarragon leaves, to serve
sea salt and freshly ground black pepper

1. Put the avocado, lemon zest and juice, mustard powder, tarragon and a grind of salt and pepper into a blender or mini chopper. Blend until smooth and creamy, adding small splashes of water to achieve the consistency of double cream.
2. Spoon the avocado dressing into a bowl, add the chicken and mix well. Check the seasoning, adding more salt and pepper if necessary.
3. Make the salad by combining the rocket, spring onion, cucumber and shredded lettuce, then pile on to a serving dish. Top with the creamy tarragon chicken and finish with a few tarragon leaves scattered over the top.

TIP: *Tarragon has a strong aniseed flavour and can be an acquired taste; you can replace it with fresh basil or chives.*

SMOKED HADDOCK & WILTED GREENS

A simple, delicious and highly nutritious breakfast, perfect for lazy Sunday mornings. The delicate chard is jam-packed with nutrients, vitamins and minerals, while the high-quality protein of the fish will keep you full until lunch.

SERVES 2
PREP: 5 MINUTES
COOK: 10 MINUTES

200g smoked haddock, preferably undyed
1 bay leaf
4 peppercorns
20g spring onion, finely sliced
1 garlic clove, finely sliced
180g rainbow chard, roughly chopped
a squeeze of lemon juice
fresh snipped chives, to serve
sea salt and freshly ground black pepper

1. Place the haddock in a pan with the bay leaf and peppercorns. Add just enough cold water to cover the fish. Cover with a lid and bring to a very gentle simmer. Poach the fish for 6–8 minutes, depending on the thickness. It's cooked when the flesh becomes opaque and flakes easily.
2. Discard the bay leaf and peppercorns and drain the fish on kitchen paper.
3. Meanwhile, over a medium heat, cook the spring onion and garlic in a splash of water for 1–2 minutes.
4. Add the chard, salt and pepper and cook for about 3–4 minutes until the chard is tender and the leaves have wilted.
5. Serve the fish on a bed of chard and add a squeeze of lemon, some black pepper and the chives.

VARIATION
- If you can't find rainbow chard, you can use spinach, and kippers can replace the smoked haddock.

APPLE & PUMPKIN SPICED CRUMBLE POTS

Is there anything as cosy and comforting as the smell of warm apples and spices on a cold day? These little pots are naturally sweet, with a gorgeous caramel note that is flavoured with warming nutmeg and ginger. Keeping some of the apple pieces whole adds a little bite, as do the earthily crunchy walnuts infused with cinnamon. These sweetly spiced pots are fantastic with a cup of bitter black coffee.

SERVES 2
PREP: 10 MINUTES
COOK: 60 MINUTES

2 medium-sized eating apples, cored and chopped
3 tbsp cold water
½ tsp ground ginger
½ tsp ground nutmeg
2 whole cloves
200g pumpkin or butternut squash, peeled, seeds removed and flesh chopped
1 tsp cinnamon
70g walnuts, finely chopped

1. Preheat the oven to 180°C/160°C fan/gas mark 4. You will need two small ovenproof ramekin dishes to serve.
2. Put the chopped apple in an ovenproof dish and sprinkle with the cold water, followed by the ginger, nutmeg and cloves. Cover tightly with foil and bake for 40 minutes until the apple is tender. Remove the cloves and allow the apple to cool.
3. Steam the pumpkin or roast it sprinkled with a splash of water in a covered dish for 20 minutes until soft.
4. Blitz the cooked pumpkin in a food processor with half the apples and their cooking juices. Divide the purée between two ramekins and top with the remaining apple pieces.
5. Stir the cinnamon through the chopped walnuts and sprinkle over the top of each ramekin.
6. Bake for 10 minutes, then serve hot.

TIP: *The pots can be batch cooked up to step 5 and kept in the fridge for up to 5 days to be baked fresh for a hot, delicious breakfast.*

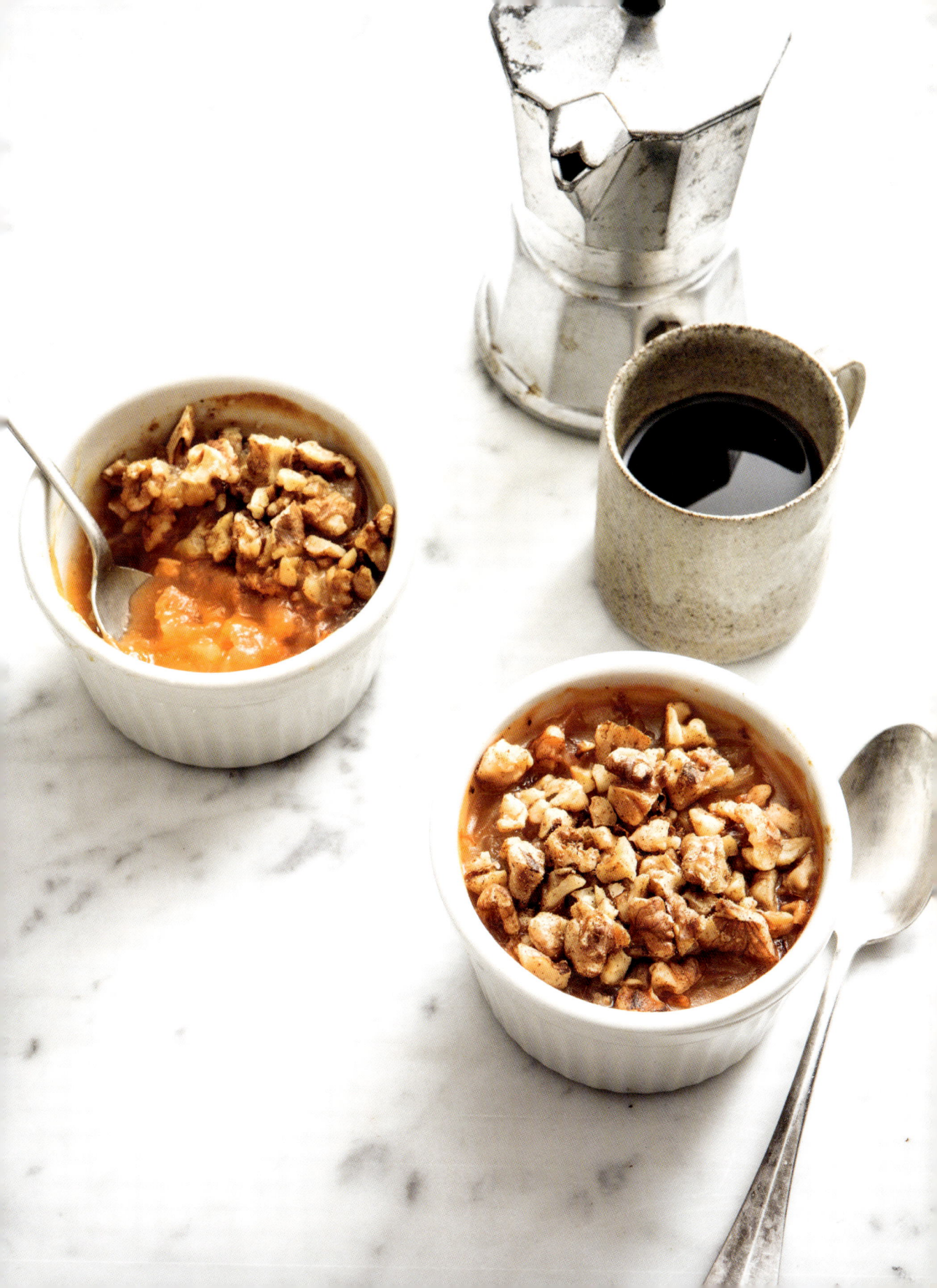

SMOKY TOFU HASH

Nutritionally, tofu is the best plant-based protein we can eat; it's almost entirely flavourless, making it a very versatile ingredient. To date, this is my hands-down, absolute favourite tofu creation. It is so moreish, evoking memories of crispy smoked bacon and my mum's Boxing Day bubble and squeak. It may not be the prettiest dish, but it is a comforting combination of fabulous earthy, smoky and sweet flavours.

SERVES 2
PREP: 10 MINUTES
COOK: 25 MINUTES

30g onion, finely diced
60g butternut squash, peeled, seeds removed and flesh finely diced
200ml fresh chicken or vegetable stock
200g firm, smoked organic tofu, finely diced
2 garlic cloves, peeled and crushed
10g/2 tsp tomato purée*
½ tsp smoked paprika*
100g Swiss chard, green cabbage or Brussels sprouts, chopped
1 tbsp chopped fresh parsley
sea salt and freshly ground black pepper

1. Cook the onion and butternut squash in a splash of stock in a shallow non-stick pan over a low to medium heat for about 5 minutes.
2. Add the tofu, garlic, tomato purée, smoked paprika and the rest of the stock. Simmer for 5 minutes, then add the Swiss chard (or other green vegetable, if using) and cook for a further 5–6 minutes until all the stock has evaporated. Season with a grind of salt and pepper.
3. Using a spatula, press the mixture down in the pan to form a flat cake. After a few minutes it will form a crust on the bottom. Stir to scrape up all the yummy chewy bits, patting the mixture back down as you go. Repeat this process 2 or 3 times until the hash is a combination of soft and crisp; this will take about 10 minutes.
4. Throw in the fresh parsley, season with salt and pepper and give the hash one final stir before plating and eating immediately.

VARIATION
- You can replace the tomato purée with an additional 10g butternut squash and the smoked paprika with a pinch of white pepper if you are avoiding nightshades.

SPINACH & MUSHROOM WRAPS

These vibrant spinach wraps are soft and springy. Here they are stuffed with mushrooms but you can ring the changes and fill them with any vegetables or salads you like. They make a great packed lunch: leave them to cool, then wrap them in greaseproof paper or foil and pop them in the fridge. Use within 24 hours.

SERVES 2
PREP: 10 MINUTES
COOK: 15 MINUTES

FOR THE WRAPS
4 eggs
100g spinach, washed
sea salt and freshly ground black pepper

FOR THE FILLING
100g king oyster mushrooms, shredded lengthways
1 garlic clove, crushed
sea salt and freshly ground black pepper

1. Preheat the oven to 150°C/130°C fan/gas mark 2.
2. Crack the eggs into a blender, add the spinach and a grind of salt and pepper, then purée until smooth.
3. Pour the spinach and egg mixture onto a non-stick baking sheet in a thin layer using a spatula to create a rough oblong shape. The mixture will be runny, so don't worry about making it perfect.
4. Bake for 12–15 minutes until the wrap is completely set. It will feel springy to the touch. Cut the cooked wrap into 2 pieces.
5. For the filling, cook the mushrooms in a non-stick frying pan for 5 minutes over a medium heat, then add the garlic and a pinch of salt and pepper. Continue to cook until the moisture from the mushrooms has evaporated and the edges are slightly burnished.
6. Assemble the wraps: spoon the mushrooms two-thirds of the way down and across the width of each wrap, then roll it up. Slice and serve hot.

TIP: *I use Bake-O-Glide to line the baking sheet. It is non-stick and makes the rolling up process very easy.*

ASPARAGUS, COURGETTE & HERB FRITTATA

A frittata is a baked omelette, similar to a crustless quiche. It is amazingly versatile; you can play around with the vegetables, herbs and spices and it tastes good hot or cold. A frittata is ideal cooked in advance – leave it to cool, then slice and eat on the go or include it as part of a packed lunch.

SERVES 2
PREP: 10 MINUTES
COOK: 10 MINUTES

4 eggs
90g fine asparagus spears, halved
70g courgette, thinly sliced
40g spring onion, finely sliced
1 tsp finely chopped fresh flat-leaf parsley
1 tsp finely chopped fresh chives
sea salt and freshly ground black pepper

1. Preheat the oven to 190°C/170°C fan/gas mark 5.
2. In a bowl, whisk the eggs and season well with salt and pepper before adding the asparagus, courgette, spring onion, parsley and chives.
3. Pour the mixture into a non-stick ovenproof pan or dish about 20cm wide.
4. Bake in the oven for 10 minutes until the eggs are fully set.

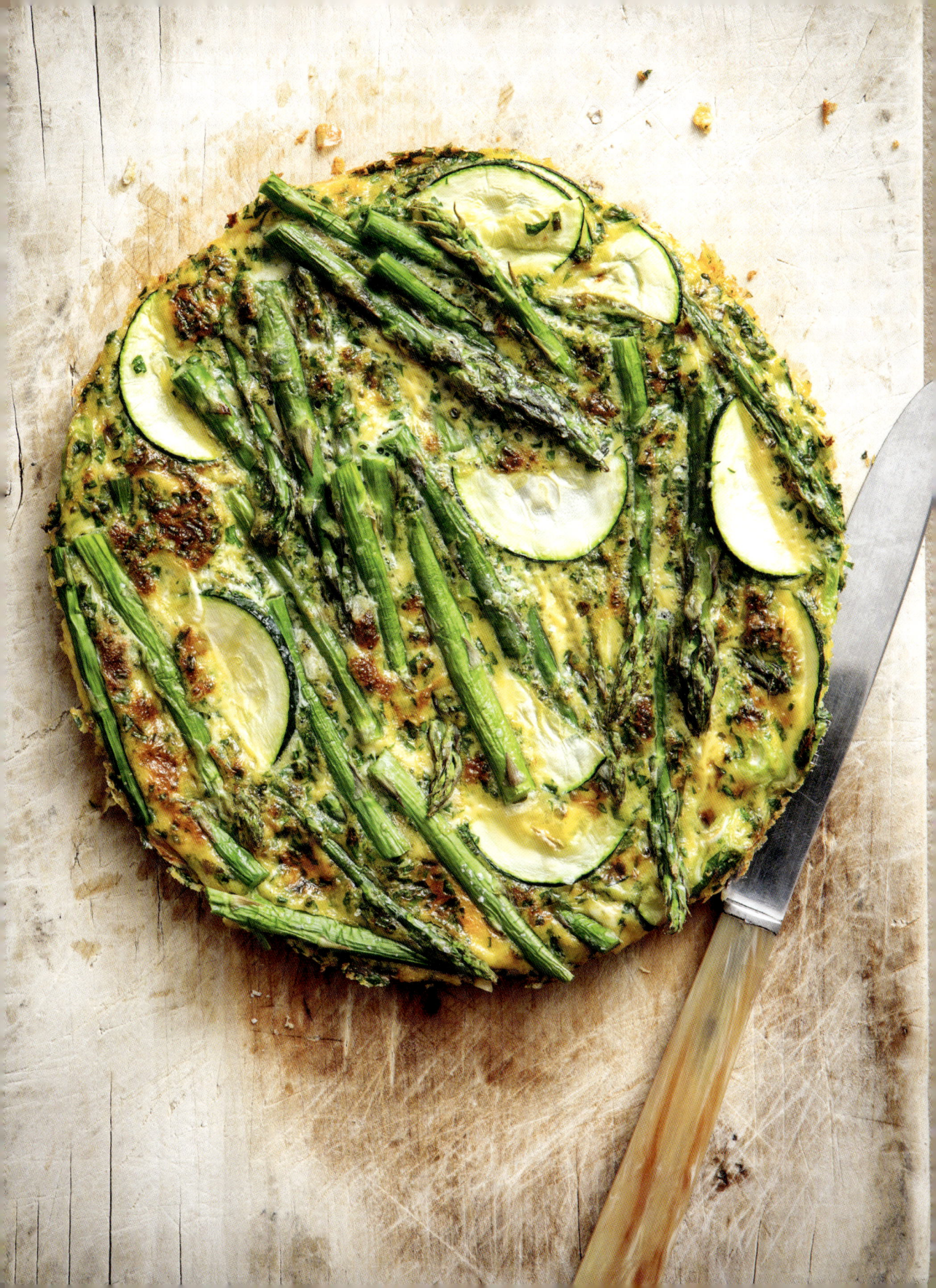

CARROT & GINGER MUFFINS

There are many variations of the HBD muffin on social media. I've tried them all and taste tested them on my discerning teenagers; here is my version. Fiery, warming ginger and sweet carrot have long been a match made in heaven; who doesn't love carrot cake? Everyone agreed that ginger tastes much more at home in this sweetly savoury eggy muffin than other spices such as cinnamon or nutmeg. The courgette gives the muffins a soft texture; without it they can be a little too springy, verging on rubbery. The vanilla doesn't overwhelm; it is there to encourage the sweet flavour of the apple to shine. The muffins keep in the fridge for 2–3 days and freeze well.

SERVES 2
PREP: 10 MINUTES

2 apples, grated
100g carrot, finely grated
100g courgette, grated
4 eggs
½ tsp pure vanilla (see Tip)
1 tsp ground ginger
pinch of sea salt

1. Preheat the oven to 190°C/170°C fan/gas mark 5.
2. Tip the grated apple, carrot and courgette on to 3 or 4 sheets of kitchen paper (or a clean tea towel) and squeeze as much moisture from them as possible.
3. Whisk the eggs, vanilla, ginger and a pinch of salt together in a bowl.
4. Add the grated apple and vegetables and stir well.
5. Divide the mixture between 4 silicone muffin cases.
6. Bake for 10 minutes, then remove the muffins from the cases, turn them upside down and bake them for a further 2 minutes.
7. Leave to cool slightly before serving.

TIP: We use 100% organic Madagascan vanilla powder by Zest & Zing. It is worth investing in a jar; a little goes a long way and it is wonderful as a sweetener for coffee or sprinkled on yoghurt or stewed apples. Alternatively, use the seeds from a vanilla pod. Slit the pod lengthways and use a sharp knife to extract the seeds.

BAKED GREEN EGGS

A perfect HBD breakfast, full of vegetables and protein and bursting with flavour. These baked pots are a cross between a shakshuka and French *oeufs en cocotte*. This is a simple way to cook eggs without oil in Phase 2. You can batch cook the veggies in advance to save time in the morning, then crack in your eggs and bake. This is an easy way to include four different veggies, herbs and spices into your breakfast – and your gut will love you for it.

SERVES 2
PREP: 10 MINUTES
COOK: 10 MINUTES

40g leek, chopped
20g spring onion, finely chopped
70g broccoli, finely chopped
70g green cabbage, finely chopped
1 small garlic clove, crushed
2 tsp tamari
a splash of water
1 tsp chopped fresh tarragon
4 eggs
chopped fresh parsley, to serve
sea salt and freshly ground black pepper

1. Preheat the oven to 200°C/180°C fan/gas mark 6.
2. In a small lidded pan, cook the leek, spring onion, broccoli, cabbage, garlic and tamari with a splash of water. Once the mixture starts bubbling, cover the pan and cook over a low heat for 5–7 minutes until everything is soft.
3. Remove from the heat and add the tarragon and a generous grind of black pepper.
4. Transfer to a small ovenproof dish. Create four wells in the vegetable mixture with a spoon and carefully crack an egg into each well.
5. Bake for about 6–10 minutes, depending on how runny you like your eggs.
6. Eat immediately sprinkled with fresh parsley and more black pepper.

> **VARIATIONS**
> - Use any green vegetables you have: Brussels sprouts, asparagus and courgettes all work well.
> - The tarragon has a distinct aniseed flavour; if that's not for you, use chives.

PHASE 2

Main Meals

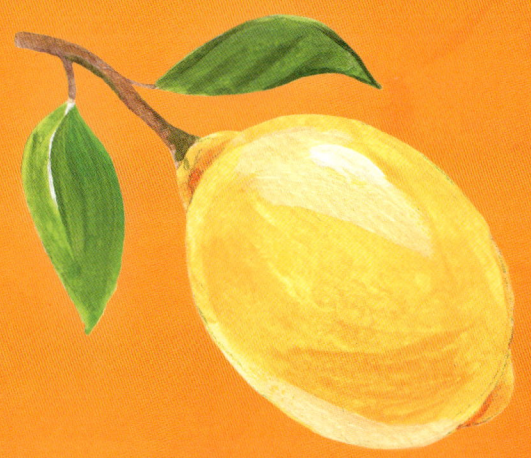

The Classics

CABBAGE LEAF GYOZAS

Our version of this Asian favourite uses tender Savoy cabbage leaves as wrappers and has a classic pork, ginger and garlic filling. The gyozas are gently poached in stock, which reduces to become a sticky, umami-rich glaze.

SERVES 2
PREP: 10 MINUTES
COOK: 10 MINUTES

180g large Savoy cabbage leaves, thick central stalk removed
260g pork mince
50g mushrooms, finely diced
30g shallots, finely diced
2 garlic cloves, crushed
1 tsp grated root ginger
1 tbsp tamari
200ml chicken stock
freshly ground white pepper

TIP: You can make the gyozas in advance up to step 4 of the recipe. Keep them covered in the fridge or freezer then cook to order. Defrost thoroughly before cooking.

1. Blanch the cabbage leaves by boiling in a saucepan of water for 3–4 minutes, then immerse them in cold water to stop the cooking process. Pat dry with kitchen paper; the leaves should now be soft and pliable.
2. Combine the pork mince, mushrooms, shallots, garlic, ginger, tamari and a pinch of white pepper in a bowl.
3. Lay the leaves flat and put 2 tablespoons of filling in the centre of each leaf (the amount will depend on the size of the leaf).
4. Tuck the top edge of the leaf over the mince and fold the sides inwards to create a triangular parcel like a samosa.
5. In a large non-stick frying pan, heat a splash of the stock and add the gyozas in a single layer with the folded side down. Cook for 1–2 minutes to seal the edges before adding the remainder of the stock.
6. Cover the pan with a lid and simmer gently over a low heat for 10–15 minutes.
7. Remove the lid and cook for a further 15 minutes until the stock has reduced to a sticky glaze.

KEDGEREE

Smoked haddock and sweet leeks, fragrant with gentle curry spices and cardamom. This kedgeree made with cauliflower rice is bursting with classic, tried and tested flavours. Green beans and a squeeze of lemon bring a fresh element. This is made on repeat in our house.

SERVES 2
PREP: 10 MINUTES
COOK: 20 MINUTES

260g smoked haddock (preferably undyed)
20g onion, finely chopped
2 garlic cloves, thinly sliced
40g leek, finely sliced
40g green beans, cut into 1–2cm pieces
4 cardamom pods, crushed
2 level tsp mild curry powder
160g cauliflower rice (see page 140)
fresh parsley and lemon juice, to serve
sea salt and freshly ground black pepper

1. Preheat the oven to 180°C/160°C fan/gas mark 4.
2. Place the haddock in an ovenproof dish with a generous splash (about 100ml) of cold water – the water creates a fish stock and adds flavour to the dish.
3. Poach in the oven for 15 minutes.
4. Meanwhile, gently cook the onion, garlic, leek and beans in a splash of water for about 5 minutes until soft.
5. Add the cardamom and curry powder and continue to cook for a few more minutes.
6. Remove the fish from the oven.
7. Add 3–4 tablespoons of the fish cooking liquid to the spicy vegetables. Add the cauliflower rice and simmer for 1–2 minutes.
8. Flake the fish and add to the cauliflower rice and vegetables. Stir gently and continue to cook for a further 1–2 minutes. Check the seasoning and add a pinch of salt if necessary.
9. To serve, sprinkle with a little parsley, a generous grind of black pepper and a good squeeze of lemon juice.

TIP: *Some smoked haddock contains more salt than others; always taste before adding additional salt.*

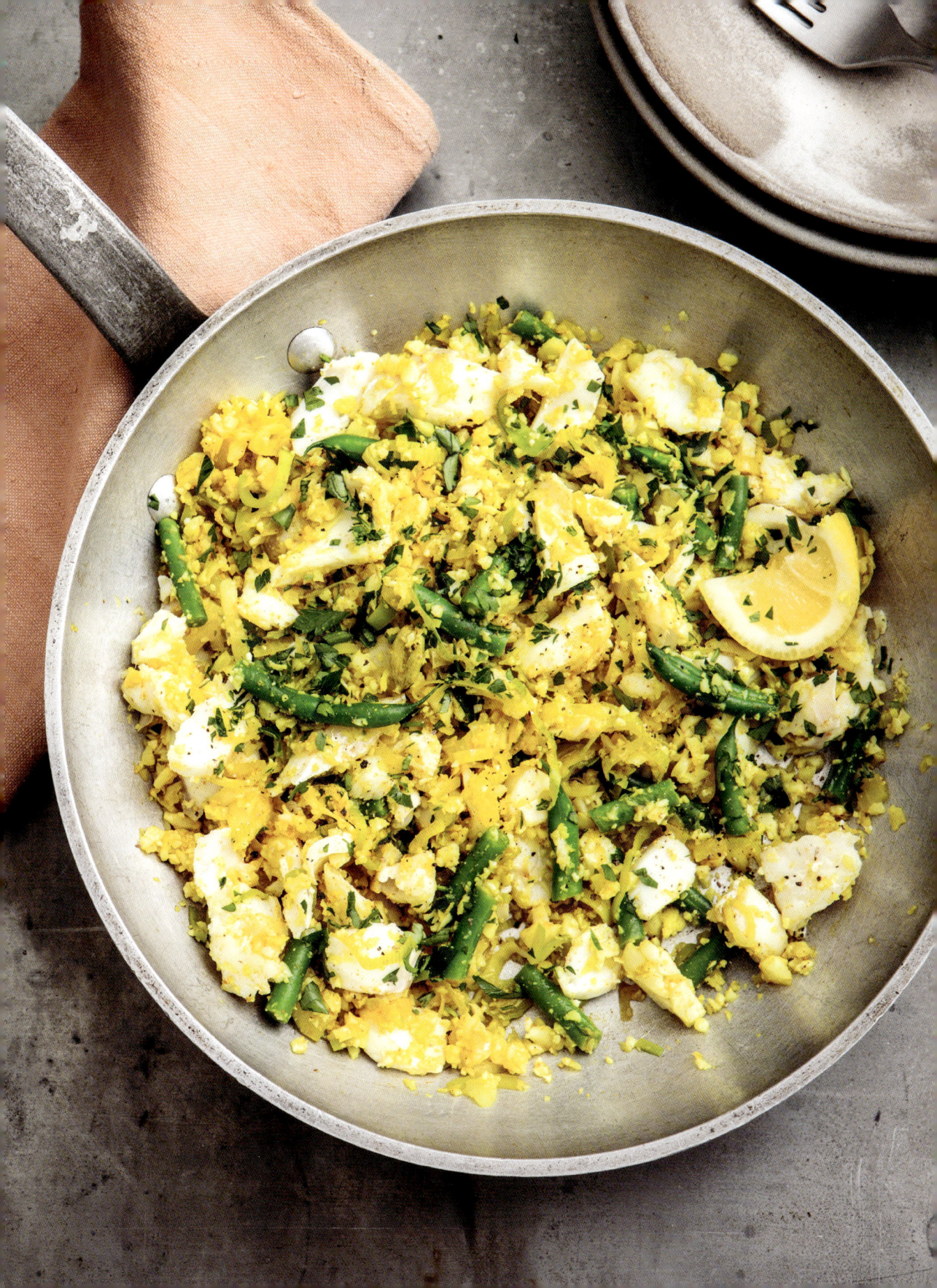

CRISPY FISH TACOS WITH SPICY GUACAMOLE

These little tacos pack a punch: they're spicy, creamy, zesty and incredibly crisp. Sea bass is the perfect fish for tacos – the fish skin crisps up brilliantly in a hot oven, leaving the flesh soft and delicious. Shredded cabbage dressed in lemon juice and sea salt balances out the cool, creamy guacamole with its sweet onion and chilli heat. Serve with a flourish of fresh coriander; you will have a fabulous combination of textures, temperatures and flavours in every bite.

SERVES 2
PREP: 20 MINUTES
COOK: 6–7 MINUTES

FOR THE TACOS
260g sea bass fillet, skin on, cut into 1–2cm strips
1 tsp smoked paprika* (optional)
a pinch of cayenne pepper* or chilli flakes* (optional)
40g red cabbage, finely sliced
a squeeze of lemon juice
80g whole baby gem lettuce leaves
sea salt

FOR THE GUACAMOLE
90g ripe avocado
30g red onion, finely chopped
20g tomato*, very finely chopped
a squeeze of lemon juice
a pinch of chilli flakes* (optional)
fresh coriander, to serve
sea salt and freshy ground black pepper

1. Preheat the oven to 220°C/200°C fan/gas mark 7.
2. Sprinkle the sea bass skin with salt, paprika and cayenne or chilli flakes (if using). Roast, skin side up, in the preheated oven for 5–6 minutes until the skin is crisp.
3. Dress the cabbage with a squeeze of lemon juice and a pinch of sea salt.
4. To make the guacamole, mash the avocado with the onion, tomato, lemon juice, chilli flakes (if using), a pinch of sea salt and a grind of black pepper. Add a splash of cold water to loosen and stir well.
5. Divide the guacamole between the baby gem leaves, top with the hot crisp fish, the cabbage and a generous scattering of fresh coriander.

VARIATION
- If you are avoiding nightshades, replace the paprika and cayenne with white pepper in the tacos. Replace the tomatoes and chilli in the guacamole with extra avocado and onion.

TIPS: Dial the heat up or down by adjusting the chilli to your taste. For extra crispy skin cook the fish skin side up in an air fryer for 4-5 minutes on high.

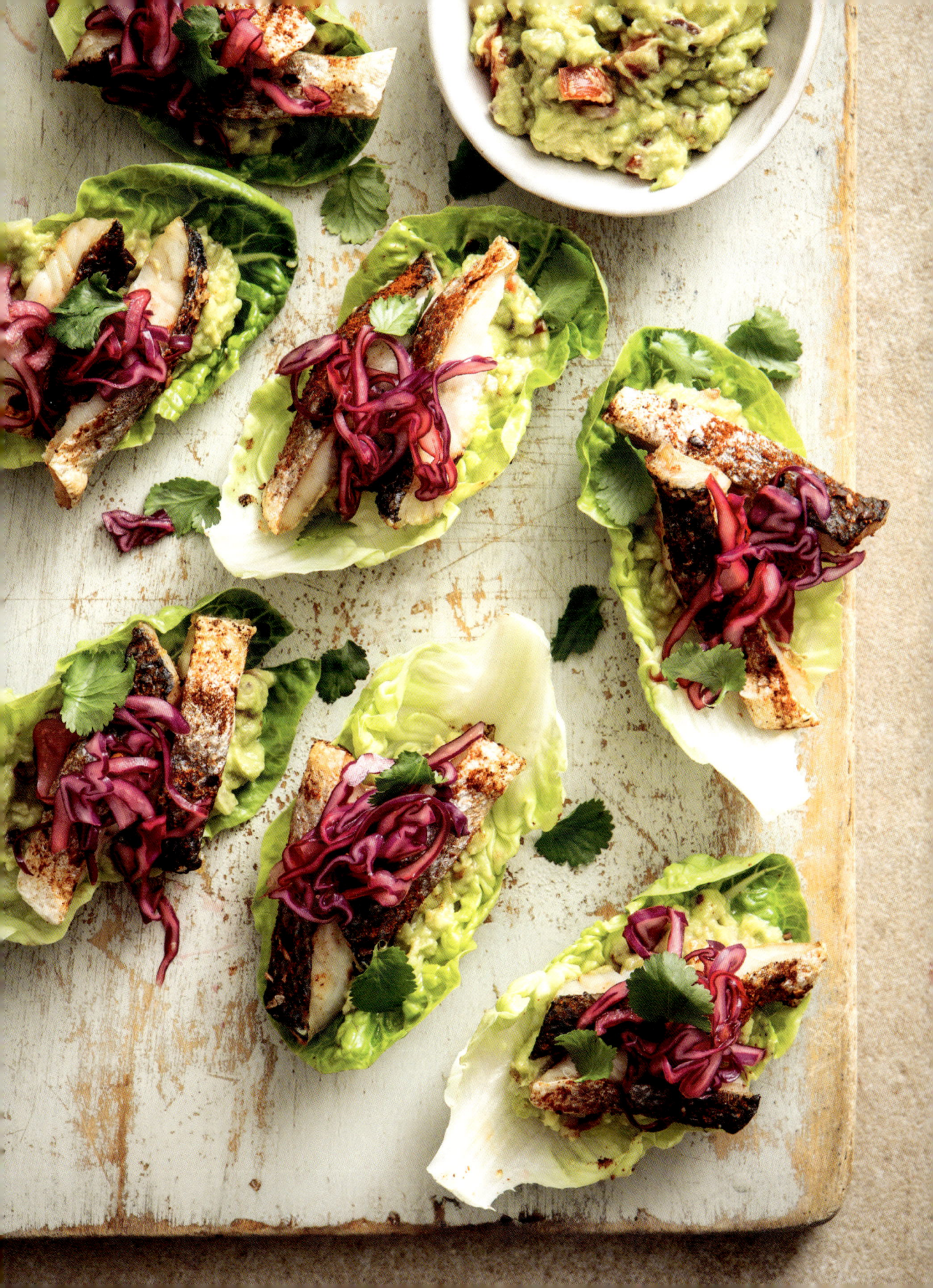

SMASH BURGERS WITH FONDANT ONION

A smash burger is thinner than a regular burger, making it quicker and easier to cook without oil; perfect for Phase 2. It is so easy to make: simply flatten the burger mixture and cook in a splash of stock. Cooking it this way keeps the burger nice and juicy. The addition of the sweet, caramelised onion fondant – so reminiscent of fried onions – and the sliced tomato gives authentic classic burger flavours.

SERVES 2
PREP: 10 MINUTES
COOK: 25 MINUTES

100g onion, in two 50g slices
260g lean minced beef
2 tbsp tamari
2 garlic cloves, crushed
2 tbsp finely chopped fresh parsley
1 tsp onion salt
splash of stock
80g asparagus tips
60g green beans
10g tomato, very finely sliced*
sea salt and freshly ground black pepper

1. Preheat the oven to 190°C/170°C fan/gas mark 5.
2. Lay the slices of onion in a small ovenproof dish and add enough cold water to almost cover them, leaving the top of the slices uncovered. Sprinkle with sea salt and bake for 20–25 minutes until tender.
3. Make the burger mixture by combining the mince, tamari, garlic, parsley, onion salt and a good grind of black pepper in a bowl. Flatten the mixture to make 2 round patties about 1cm thick.
4. Pour a splash of stock into a non-stick frying pan, add the burgers and cook over a medium heat for 3–4 minutes. Flip the burgers over and cook for a few more minutes until they are cooked through and the stock has evaporated.
5. Meanwhile, steam or boil the asparagus and beans together for 3–4 minutes.
6. Serve the burgers topped with the tomato and onion with the beans and asparagus alongside.

> **TIPS:** *If you are avoiding nightshades, replace the tomato with an extra 10g of beans or asparagus. These burgers are delicious served with Red Pepper Ketchup (see page 56).*

JAMBALAYA

Jambalaya is a Cajun rice dish that originated in Louisiana. It is quite literally a jumble of smoky, spicy, savoury and sweet flavours. Our HBD version hits all the right notes: sweet butternut is balanced with smoky spices, and the fresh tomato and pepper are delicious with the nutty lentil rice. I love chickpea and lentil rice; both have a firm bite and taste a little like orzo pasta. The lentil version here looks pretty with the red spices and vegetables, but use chickpea rice if that's what you have. Jambalaya is a satisfying and filling Phase 2 dish, perfect for days when you're feeling extra hungry. This recipe is not suitable for those avoiding nightshades.

SERVES 2
PREP: 5 MINUTES
COOK: 20 MINUTES

80g red onion, very finely chopped
300ml chicken or vegetable stock
3 garlic cloves, finely sliced
60g butternut squash, peeled snd finely diced
80g red pepper*, finely chopped
40g tomato*, finely chopped
2 tsp smoked paprika*
½ tsp chilli flakes*
160g lentil rice
200ml boiling water
fresh parsley to serve
sea salt and freshly ground black pepper

1. Gently cook the red onion in a splash of stock for 2–3 minutes to soften.
2. Add the garlic, butternut squash, pepper, tomato, spices and lentil rice and cook for 1–2 minutes, ensuring that the rice is well coated with the spices.
3. Add the remaining stock, the boiling water and a grind of salt and pepper. Increase the heat slightly and continue to cook for 15 minutes, stirring occasionally. Most of the liquid will evaporate, but if it hasn't, turn up the heat and cook for a further minute or two. Test that the rice is cooked; it should be al dente. Be careful not to overcook it.
4. Check the seasoning, adding more salt and pepper if necessary.
5. Serve with a flourish of fresh parsley.

TIP: *Will keep in the fridge for 2–3 days and freezes well.*

KING PRAWN PAELLA

The classic Spanish flavours of saffron and smoked paprika with plump, sweet prawns will transport you back to holidays in the sunshine. Cauliflower rice has little or no flavour and soaks up the golden hues and flavours of the spices brilliantly. This recipe was taste-tested by my Spanish friend, who gave it her stamp of approval as an authentic, healthy version of the iconic national dish. Unless you are pescatarian, I recommend using a good chicken stock to add the meaty depth of flavour you get in a traditional mixed seafood and chicken paella.

SERVES 2
PREP: 10 MINUTES
COOK: 15 MINUTES

20g shallot, very finely chopped
30g red pepper*, chopped
3 garlic cloves, very finely chopped
1 tsp smoked paprika*
200g cauliflower rice (see Tip)
200ml fresh chicken or vegetable stock
10g/2 tsp tomato purée*
a pinch of saffron strands
260g raw king prawns, shelled
lemon wedges and fresh parsley, to serve
sea salt and freshly ground black pepper

1. In a frying pan or wok, cook the shallot and red pepper in a splash of water for about 5 minutes until they are slightly softened.
2. Add the garlic and smoked paprika and cook for a further minute.
3. Add the cauliflower rice, stock, tomato purée and saffron strands and cook for 5–7 minutes until most of the stock has been absorbed. Add the prawns and a grind of salt and pepper.
4. Continue to cook for about 5 minutes until the prawns turn pink and are completely cooked through.
5. Serve scattered with fresh parsley and with a squeeze of lemon.

VARIATION
- If you are avoiding nightshades, use sliced courgette instead of red pepper and add a pinch of white pepper in place of the smoked paprika.

TIP: Cauliflower rice is readily available in shops but is also very easy to make. Remove the florets from a fresh cauliflower and use the stalks to make your rice (using just the stalks gives more texture to the rice once it's cooked). Chop the stalks into medium-sized pieces and pulse very briefly in a food processor.

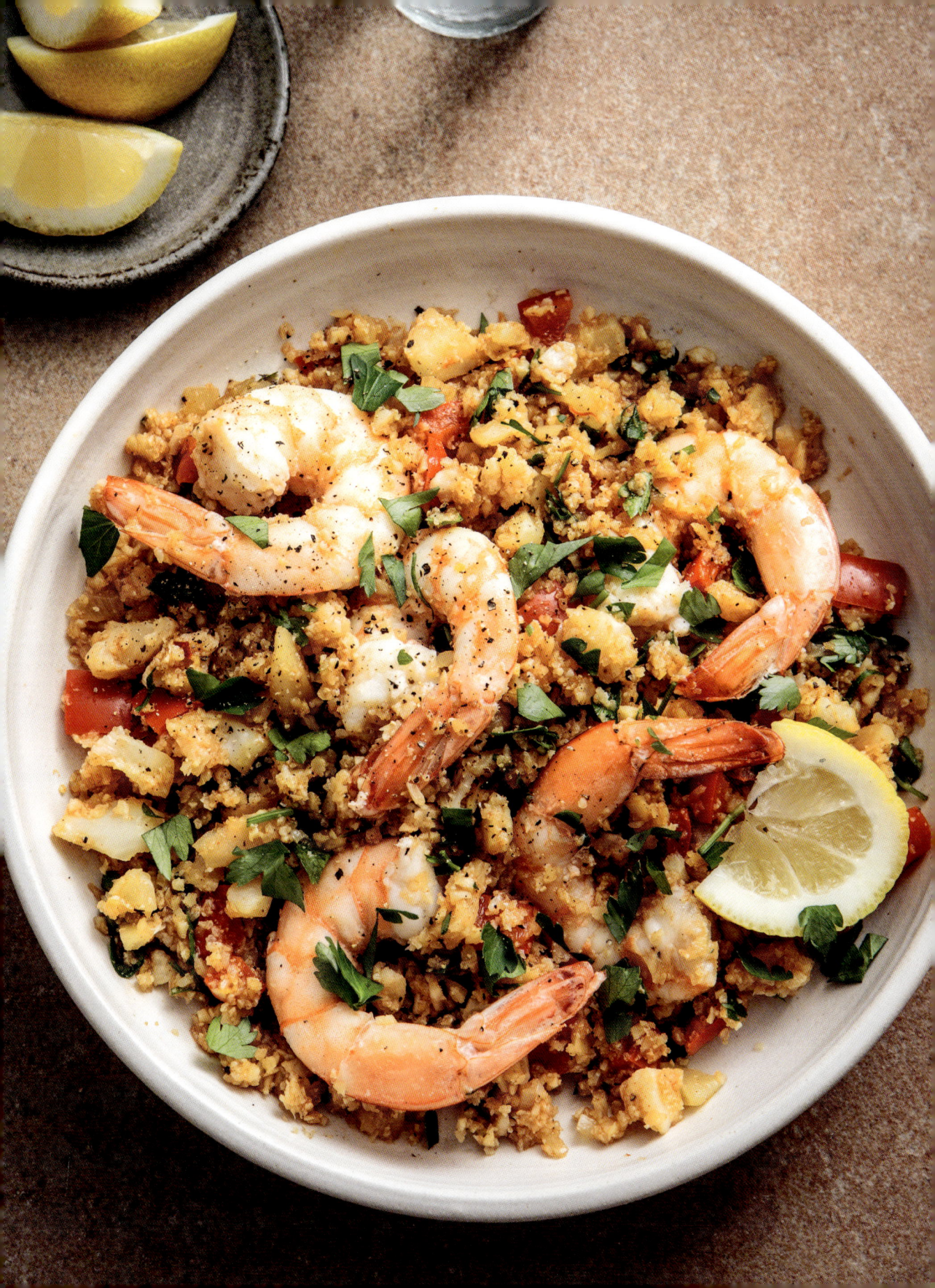

SHIITAKE MUSHROOM, SPINACH & THYME RISOTTO

Shiitake mushrooms are becoming increasingly popular and are readily available in most supermarkets. Their umami-rich flavour and firm, meaty texture make them a hero of the mushroom world. Deemed a superfood, they are packed with antioxidants and vitamins. I highly recommend the chickpea rice by Mr Organic, which has a firm bite and tastes a little like orzo pasta. The addition of woody thyme, garlic and tamari gives this dish an autumnal feel: rich, savoury and incredibly filling. It freezes well.

SERVES 2
PREP: 10 MINUTES
COOK: 20–25 MINUTES

40g shallot or onion, very finely chopped
300ml chicken or vegetable stock
3 garlic cloves, finely sliced
160g chickpea rice
150ml boiling water
1 tbsp tamari
180g shiitake mushrooms, sliced
3 sprigs of fresh thyme
40g baby spinach leaves
sea salt and freshly ground black pepper

1. In a non-stick pan or wok, gently cook the shallot for 2–3 minutes in a little stock over a low heat.
2. Add the garlic and cook for a further minute before adding the rice, the rest of the stock, the boiling water, tamari, mushrooms and thyme. Increase the heat slightly and cook for 15 minutes, stirring occasionally.
3. Add the spinach and cook for a further 2 minutes until it has wilted. Most of the liquid will have evaporated, but if some is left, turn up the heat a little and cook for a further minute or two.
4. Test that the rice is cooked; it should be al dente.
5. Season with a generous grind of black pepper and a pinch of sea salt if necessary.

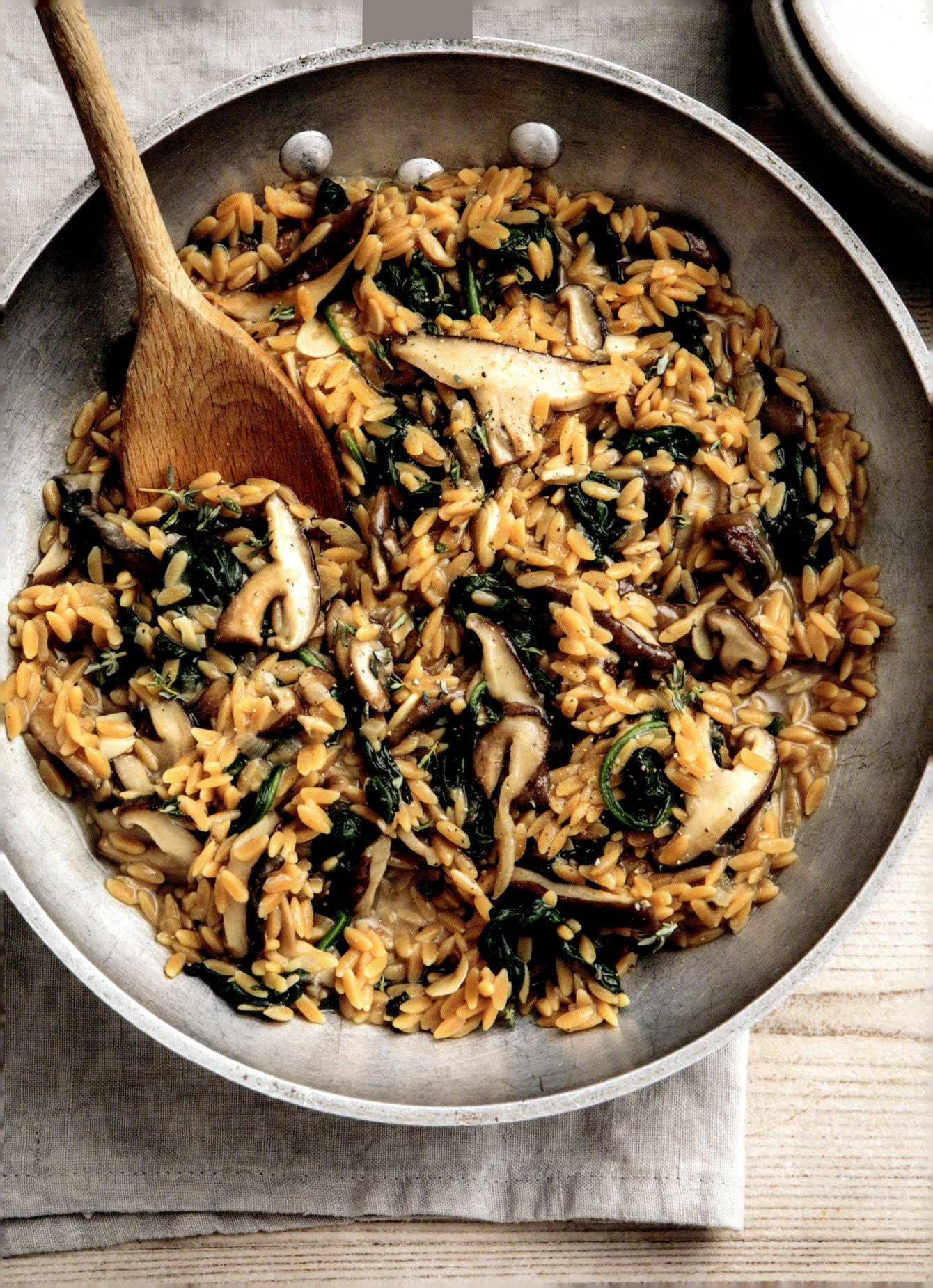

SPRING CHICKEN CASSEROLE

A simple Provençal casserole full of delicate vegetables, tender chicken and subtle flavours. Finely dicing all the vegetables allows quick cooking, resulting in a fresh tasting, light and bright taste of springtime – hence the name!

SERVES 2
PREP: 15 MINUTES
COOK: 20 MINUTES

30g onion, finely diced
30g carrot, finely sliced
30g celery, finely sliced
50g fennel, finely sliced
3 garlic cloves, finely sliced
350ml chicken stock
260g skinless chicken breasts, thinly sliced
50g green beans, finely sliced
40g courgette, finely diced
30g spring greens, sliced
a squeeze of lemon and 1 tbsp chopped fresh dill, to serve
sea salt and freshly ground white pepper

1. Put the onion, carrot, celery, fennel and garlic in a saucepan with a splash of the stock. Season with a pinch of salt and white pepper. Simmer gently for 5 minutes to soften the vegetables.
2. Add the remaining stock, the chicken, green beans, courgette and spring greens. Bring to the boil briefly, turn the heat to its lowest setting, cover the pan with a lid and simmer gently for about 2–3 minutes until the chicken is opaque and cooked through and the greens are tender and wilted.
3. Remove from the heat. Add a squeeze of lemon and some fresh dill and season with salt and pepper. The casserole will keep for 3–4 days in the fridge and freezes well.

VARIATION
- Swap the mild aniseed flavours of fennel and dill for asparagus and flat-leaf parsley.

MOUSSAKA

This is one of my favourite Greek dishes. Dry frying the lamb mince almost to the point of caramelisation creates a deep umami flavour, perfect with the woody rosemary and fragrant garlic. Apologies to purists; this moussaka contains herbs in place of the usual spices, but I promise it is delicious nevertheless! This dish freezes well.

SERVES 2
PREP: 10 MINUTES
COOK: 30 MINUTES

260g lamb mince
60g onion, finely sliced
3 garlic cloves, finely sliced
60g mushrooms, finely diced
40g courgette, halved and sliced
300ml chicken or vegetable stock
1 tbsp finely chopped fresh rosemary
100g aubergine*, finely sliced into rounds
sea salt and freshly ground white pepper

1. Preheat the oven to 190°C/170°C fan/gas mark 5.
2. Gently fry the mince in a non-stick frying pan, stirring regularly, for about 7–8 minutes until it is well cooked, deep brown and slightly caramelised at the edges.
3. Add the onion, garlic, mushrooms and a pinch of salt and pepper, and continue to cook for a few minutes until the moisture from the mushrooms has evaporated.
4. Add the courgette, stock and rosemary and simmer uncovered for 10 minutes.
5. Transfer into a small ovenproof dish and place the aubergine slices in a single layer on top. Press them gently into the mince so they are partially immersed in the sauce.
6. Bake for 25–30 minutes until the aubergine is tender and burnished.

> **VARIATION**
> - If you are avoiding nightshades, replace the aubergine with slices of courgette.

POMEGRANATE COUSCOUS

This bejewelled couscous, studded with sweet pomegranate seeds, is as versatile as it is beautiful and literally goes with anything. Broccoli stalks are miraculously transformed into a couscous-like crumb in a food processor or chopper with a few pulses. Mint and parsley bring brightness, while peppery radish adds crisp crunch. You'll want to make this couscous on repeat. This dish is a treat for your gut microbiome and is jam-packed with antioxidants, vitamins and minerals. It is delicious for breakfast too, served with toasted pumpkin seeds, or as a quick lunch served with salty feta.

SERVES 2
PREP: 15 MINUTES

160g broccoli stalks, roughly chopped
20g red onion, finely diced
30g cucumber, diced
20g radish, thinly sliced
30g cherry tomatoes*, finely chopped (optional)
100g pomegranate seeds
2 tbsp chopped fresh parsley
2 tbsp chopped fresh mint
sea salt and freshly ground black pepper

1. Briefly pulse the broccoli stalks in a food processor or chopper until you have a mixture resembling couscous.
2. Combine the broccoli couscous, onion, cucumber, radish, cherry tomatoes and pomegranate seeds in a bowl.
3. Add the parsley, mint and a generous pinch of salt and pepper and mix well.
4. Serve immediately with protein of your choice, e.g. 80g feta or 130g chicken or salmon. The couscous will keep in the fridge for up to 2 days.

VARIATION
- If you are avoiding nightshades, replace the tomato with extra radish and cucumber.

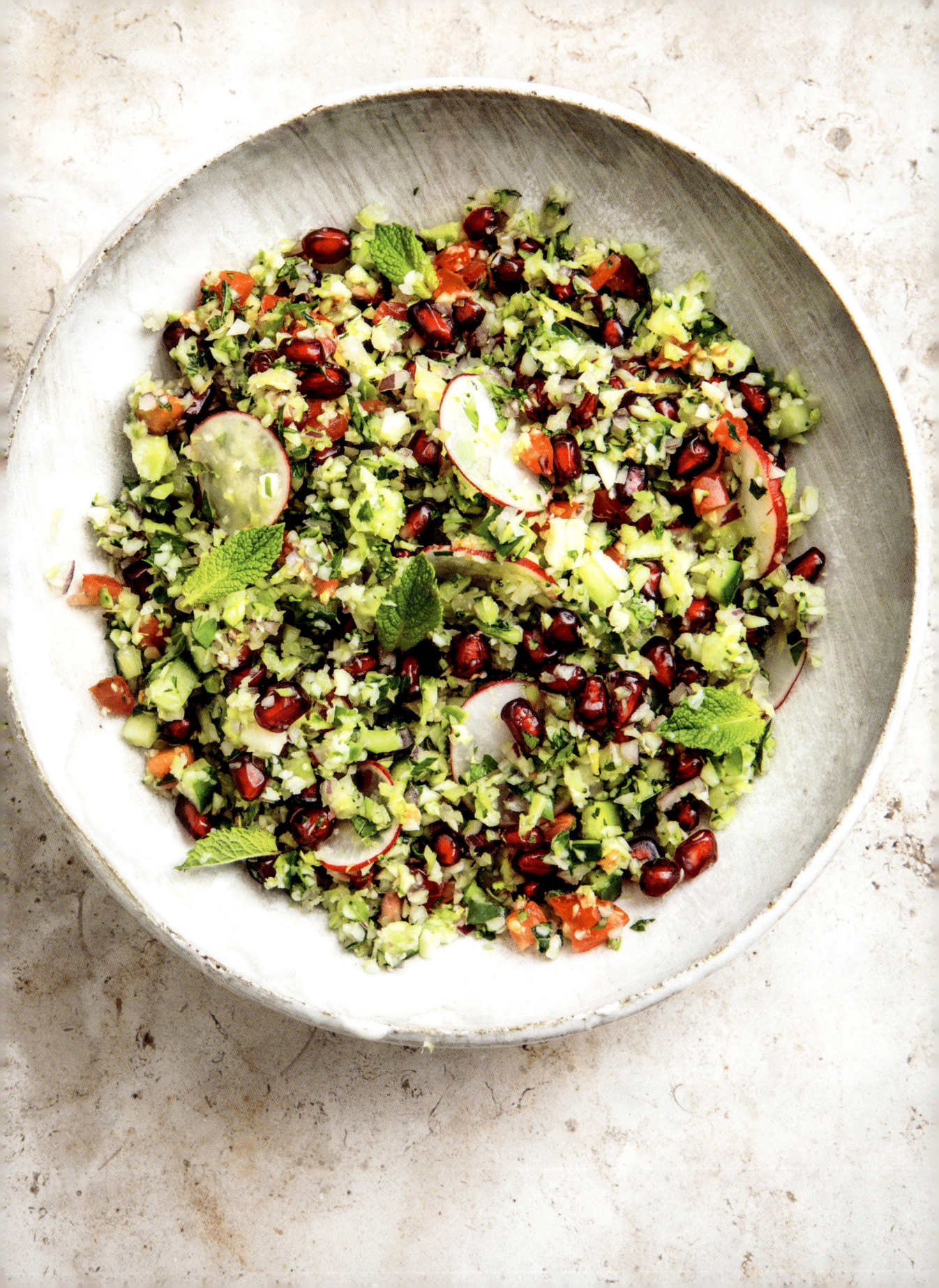

Crowd Pleasers

LAMB KOFTAS WITH BABA GANOUSH

This recipe is inspired by travels to Turkey, where I fell in love with delicious Middle Eastern spices and the abundance of fresh herbs. It's a dish of contrasting flavours, temperatures and textures. Little juicy spiced koftas packed with flavour are served hot, straight from the oven. The cool, smoky baba ganoush complements them perfectly making a glorious combination, nestled in crisp fresh lettuce. The baba ganaoush is not suitable for those avoiding nightshades.

SERVES 2
PREP: 15 MINUTES
COOK: 30 MINUTES

FOR THE BABA GANOUSH
160g aubergine*
1 large garlic clove, crushed
2 tsp lemon juice
½ tsp smoked paprika*
60g whole baby gem leaves
20g red onion, finely sliced, to serve

FOR THE KOFTAS
260g minced lamb
3 garlic cloves, crushed
1 tsp ground cumin
2 tsp ground coriander
2 tbsp finely chopped fresh mint
2 tbsp finely chopped fresh parsley
20g onion, grated
a splash of stock, for baking
sea salt and freshly ground pepper

1. Preheat the oven to 190°C/170°C fan/gas mark 5.
2. Make the baba ganoush. Halve the aubergine and lay it skin side down in an ovenproof dish, then score the flesh with 2 or 3 deep diagonal cuts. Season with a grind of salt and pepper, add a splash of water, cover with foil and bake until soft – about 40–50 minutes.
3. Allow to cool, scoop out the flesh and discard the skins.
4. Purée the aubergine flesh with the garlic, lemon juice, smoked paprika and a pinch of salt. Add a splash of cold water, if necessary, and purée until you have a smooth, silky dip. Chill.
5. For the koftas, put the mince, crushed garlic, cumin, coriander, mint, parsley, grated onion and a generous grind of salt and pepper into a bowl. Mix well to combine all the ingredients and shape into four oval patties.
6. Put a splash of stock into a shallow baking dish, add the koftas and bake until they are cooked through; this takes about 12–14 minutes.
7. Spoon the baba ganoush into the baby gem leaves and top each with a hot kofta and red onion.

TIP: The baba ganoush will keep in a sealed jar in the fridge for 3 days. Stir well before serving.

BAKED FETA PARCELS

Baked feta is salty and rich and contrasts wonderfully with the sweet, tangy pepper sauce in this recipe. Parcelling the cheese in courgette ribbons gives the dish a little bite and texture. They're easy to prepare using a potato peeler, which makes the ribbons wafer thin. This is a one-dish wonder, so easy to prepare and packed with flavour. This recipe isn't suitable for those avoiding nightshades.

SERVES 2
PREP: 20 MINUTES
COOK: 50 MINUTES

100g red pepper*, roughly chopped
30g onion, in one piece
4 garlic cloves, unpeeled
120g thin courgette ribbons
160g feta cheese, cut into six equal chunks
100ml fresh chicken or vegetable stock
10g/2 tsp tomato purée*
fresh basil leaves, to serve
sea salt and freshly ground black pepper

1. Preheat the oven to 190°C/170°C fan/gas mark 5.
2. Wrap the red pepper, onion and garlic in foil and roast for about 20–25 minutes until soft.
3. Meanwhile, divide the courgette into six equal piles.
4. Take one pile and lay 4 or 5 ribbons vertically, overlapping the edges to create a sheet. Lay 4 or 5 more ribbons horizontally on top of the first layer to create a cross shape. Place a chunk of feta in the middle of the cross and fold the courgette around the cheese to create a neat parcel. Repeat with the remaining courgette ribbons until you have 6 neat parcels.
5. Remove the vegetables from the oven and squeeze the soft garlic flesh from the papery skins. Put the roasted peppers, onions and garlic into a blender, add the stock and tomato purée and blend to make the sauce. Season with a grind of salt and pepper.
6. Pour the sauce into a small ovenproof dish. Place the feta parcels on top and bake for 25 minutes until the sauce is bubbling and the cheese is soft. Scatter with basil leaves and serve.

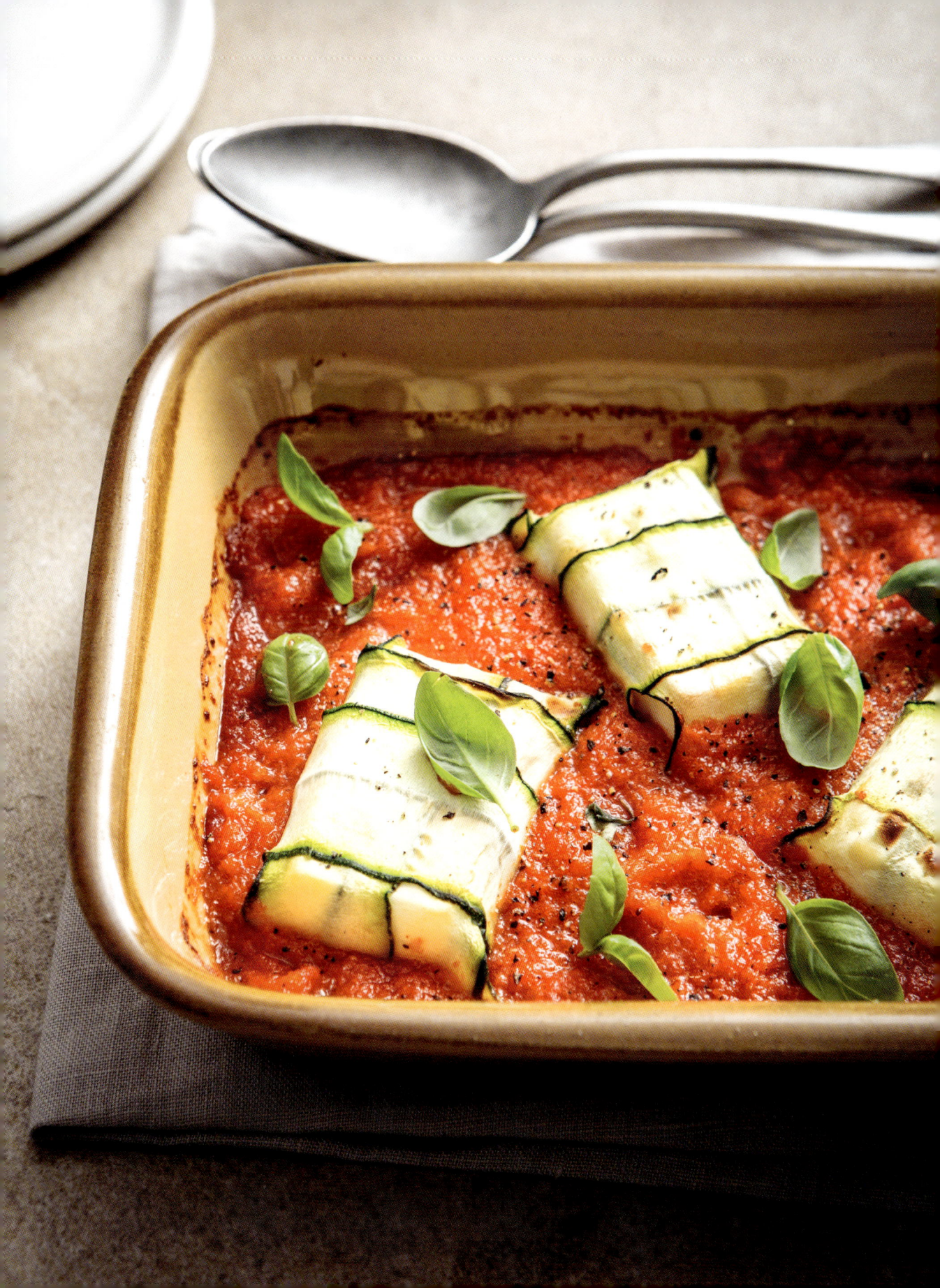

CHICKEN & POMEGRANATE TAGINE WITH SAFFRON COUSCOUS

For this reinvented HBD tagine, I've used pomegranates in place of the traditional dried apricots or dates. Most shop-bought pomegranate molasses is packed with nasties, but making a quick syrup from fresh pomegranate seeds gives a fruity, sweet note to this dish.

SERVES 2
PREP: 20 MINUTES
COOK: 20 MINUTES

50g red onion, finely sliced
350ml stock
3 garlic cloves, crushed
2 tsp ground cumin
1 tsp ground coriander
1 tsp ground ginger
260g chicken breast, sliced into 2–3cm pieces
100g butternut squash, peeled and chopped into chunks
10g/2 tsp tomato purée*
sea salt and freshly ground black pepper

FOR THE POMEGRANATE SYRUP
150g fresh pomegranate seeds
½ cinnamon stick
50g pomegranate seeds and fresh mint, to serve

FOR THE SAFFRON COUSCOUS
1 garlic clove, finely chopped
100g cauliflower rice (see page 140)
a pinch of saffron strands
1 tbsp chopped fresh parsley

1. Make the tagine in a low-sided pan over a medium heat. Cook the onion in a splash of stock for about 3–4 minutes until soft.
2. Add the garlic, cumin, ground coriander, ginger and a pinch of salt and cook for 1–2 minutes.
3. Add the chicken, butternut squash, the rest of the stock and the tomato purée and simmer uncovered over a low heat for 15–20 minutes.
4. Meanwhile, make the pomegranate syrup. Put the pomegranate seeds into a small saucepan with the cinnamon stick. Cover with 150ml cold water. Bring to the boil and simmer for 10–15 minutes. The seeds will pop slightly and the water will evaporate to leave 3–4 tablespoons of pink syrup in the pan. Remove the cinnamon stick and strain the syrup through a sieve. Push the seeds into the sieve with the back of a spoon to squeeze out the juice. Discard the seeds, then add the syrup to the tagine along with the cinnamon stick.
5. Towards the end of the tagine cooking time, make the cauliflower saffron couscous. Cook the garlic in a pan with a splash of water for 1–2 minutes. Add the cauliflower rice, saffron strands, a splash more water and a generous grind of salt and pepper. Simmer over a low heat for 3–4 minutes until the liquid has evaporated. Remove from the heat and add the fresh parsley.
6. Remove the tagine from the oven and check that the squash is tender and the chicken thoroughly cooked. Taste and add salt and pepper as necessary.
7. Serve the tagine with the couscous and scatter with the remaining pomegranate seeds and fresh mint.

CAPONATA WITH COD

Caponata is a classic warm salad of aubergine, Mediterranean vegetables, olives and capers. Traditionally served with locally caught fish, here it is baked with succulent cod. The juices and flavours of the cod combine with the salty, sweet and earthy flavours of the caponata, resulting in a rich one-pot main course, vibrant and delicious. This recipe is not suitable for those avoiding nightshades.

SERVES 2
PREP: 15 MINUTES
COOK: 30 MINUTES

40g onion, finely chopped
3 garlic cloves, crushed
120g aubergine*, roughly chopped
60g courgette, roughly chopped
30g red pepper*, roughly chopped
10g/2 tsp tomato purée*
8 black olives, halved
2 tsp capers in brine, drained
160ml boiling water
260g cod loin, cut into 2 pieces
fresh parsley and a squeeze of fresh lemon juice, to serve
sea salt and freshly ground black pepper

1. Preheat the oven to 190°C/170°C fan/gas mark 5.
2. In a deep-sided ovenproof pan, cook the onion and garlic in a splash of cold water for 5 minutes until soft.
3. Add the aubergine, courgette, pepper, tomato purée, olives, capers, boiling water and a good grind of salt and pepper. Cook over a low heat for about 10–15 minutes until the vegetables have softened.
4. Place the cod loin pieces on top of the caponata and transfer the pan to the oven to bake for 15–18 minutes, depending on the thickness of your fish. The fish is cooked when it flakes easily with a fork.
5. Taste and season with salt and pepper if necessary
6. Serve immediately sprinkled with fresh parsley and a squeeze of lemon.

TIP: *Caponata also goes brilliantly with meat, cheese and pulses.*

CRISPY SEA BASS WITH MANGO SALSA

The natural oils in sea bass help to crisp the skin under a hot grill with no need for oil, making it perfect for a speedy and delicious Phase 2 meal. Sweet juicy mango, creamy avocado and crunchy red pepper combine to create a salsa jam-packed with vibrant textures and flavours.

SERVES 2
PREP: 10 MINUTES
COOK: 10 MINUTES

FOR THE SEA BASS
260g sea bass fillets
1 tsp chilli powder* (optional)
sea salt

FOR THE SALSA
100g red pepper*, diced
40g red onion, finely diced
40g fresh tomato*, diced
80g avocado, diced
200g ripe mango, diced
1 small, mild green chilli*, chopped (optional)
2 tbsp chopped fresh coriander stalks and leaves
sea salt and freshly ground black pepper

1. Preheat the grill to high.
2. Place the sea bass fillets skin side up on a non-stick baking tray. Make 2–3 slashes in the skin and sprinkle with a pinch of sea salt and chilli powder (if using).
3. Grill the fish for 6–8 minutes until the skin blisters and crisps and the flesh flakes easily.
4. Meanwhile, make the salsa by combining all the ingredients in a bowl and seasoning with salt and pepper.
5. Spoon the salsa onto plates and top with the crispy sea bass to serve.

> **VARIATION**
> - If you are avoiding nightshades, use additional red onion and avocado in place of the pepper and tomato in the salsa.

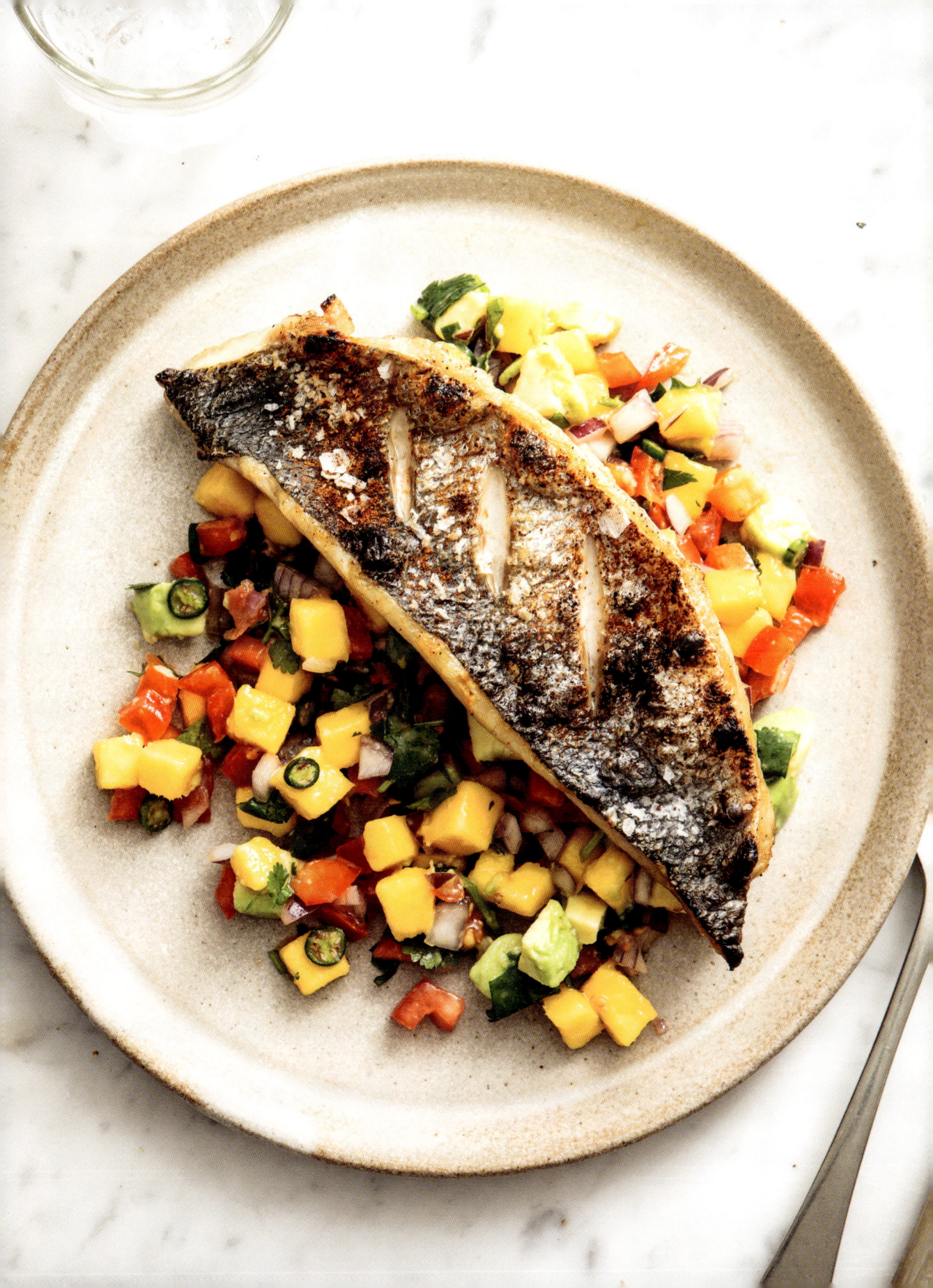

SWEET & SOUR SALMON

This HBD sweet and sour sauce is a revelation; it's just as good as the one in my local Chinese takeaway, and has none of the MSG and other nasties. The sweetness comes courtesy of the mango, cooked down to create a syrupy sauce. A splash of apple cider vinegar brings the sour flavour, and tamari, garlic and chilli give the sauce a salty, spicy depth. Serve with the addition of steamed jasmine rice for family and friends.

SERVES 2
PREP: 5 MINUTES
COOK: 15 MINUTES

60g onion, finely sliced
a splash of cold water
3 garlic cloves, finely sliced
60g carrot, finely julienned
70g green pepper* finely julienned
70g red or yellow pepper* finely julienned
160g ripe mango, chopped
2 tbsp tamari
1 red chilli* very finely chopped (optional)
2 tbsp apple cider vinegar
260g salmon, cut into 2–3cm cubes
fresh coriander, to serve (optional)

1. In a non-stick pan, cook the onion in a splash of cold water until softened. This takes about 4–5 minutes.
2. Add the garlic, carrot, peppers, mango, tamari, chilli and apple cider vinegar. Cover the pan with a lid and cook over a gentle heat for 5–6 minutes until the vegetables have softened and the mango has begun to break down.
3. Add the salmon pieces and continue to cook uncovered for 5–6 minutes, until the flesh is opaque and the sauce has thickened to a syrupy consistency.
4. Serve immediately with a flourish of fresh coriander (if using).

VARIATIONS
- Delicious made with prawns, tofu, chicken or pork. Follow the method above and add your protein of choice, ensuring that it is thoroughly cooked through before serving.
- Use courgette batons in place of peppers if you are avoiding nightshades.

TIP: *Dial the heat up or down by adjusting the amount of chilli.*

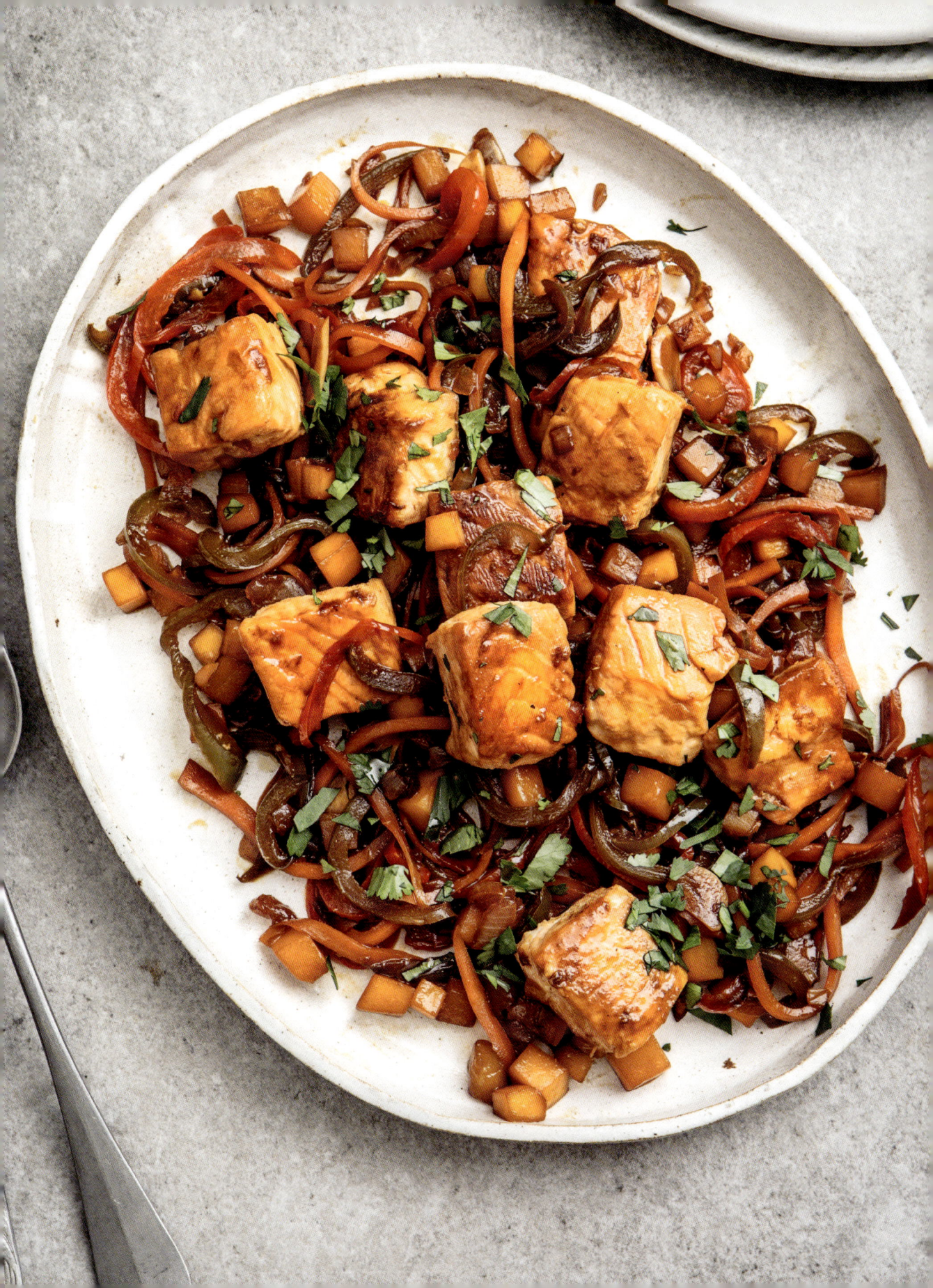

CHICKEN SHAWARMA WITH GREEK SALAD

The Middle East meets the southern Mediterranean in this recipe. The succulent kebab is fragrant, with warm notes of cumin and the fruity flavours and gentle heat of baharat, also known as Lebanese 7 spice.

SERVES 2
PREP: 20 MINUTES
(PLUS 20–60 MINUTES MARINADING)
COOK: 20 MINUTES

FOR THE SHAWARMA
zest and juice of 1 lemon
½ tsp ground cumin
½ tsp baharat/Lebanese 7 spice*
2 garlic cloves, crushed
260g skinless chicken breast, cut into cubes
sea salt and freshly ground black pepper

FOR THE GREEK SALAD
150g cucumber, deseeded, peeled and roughly chopped
50g red pepper*, roughly chopped
40g cherry tomatoes*, chopped
20g red onion, sliced
8 black olives, halved
a squeeze of lemon juice
a pinch of dried oregano
sea salt and freshly ground black pepper

1. Make the marinade for the chicken by combining the lemon zest and juice, the spices, garlic and a good grind of salt and pepper in a bowl.
2. Add the chicken pieces to the marinade and turn to coat them evenly. Cover and leave to infuse for about 20–60 minutes in the fridge.
3. If you are using wooden skewers, soak them in water for at least 20 minutes to prevent them burning.
4. When you are ready to cook the kebabs, preheat the oven to 190°C/170°C fan/gas mark 5.
5. Thread the chicken onto the skewers and roast for 15–20 minutes, turning once halfway through cooking.
6. Meanwhile, assemble the salad. Mix the cucumber, red pepper, tomato, red onion and black olives in a bowl. Add the lemon juice, a grind of salt and pepper and stir well. Sprinkle with oregano to serve.
7. Remove the kebabs from the oven and check that they are thoroughly cooked and the juices run clear. Serve alongside the Greek salad.

VARIATIONS
- If you are avoiding nightshades, replace the pepper and tomatoes with radish and celery.
- Baharat contains a small amount of paprika; you can replace it with a pinch of cinnamon, ground coriander and white pepper.

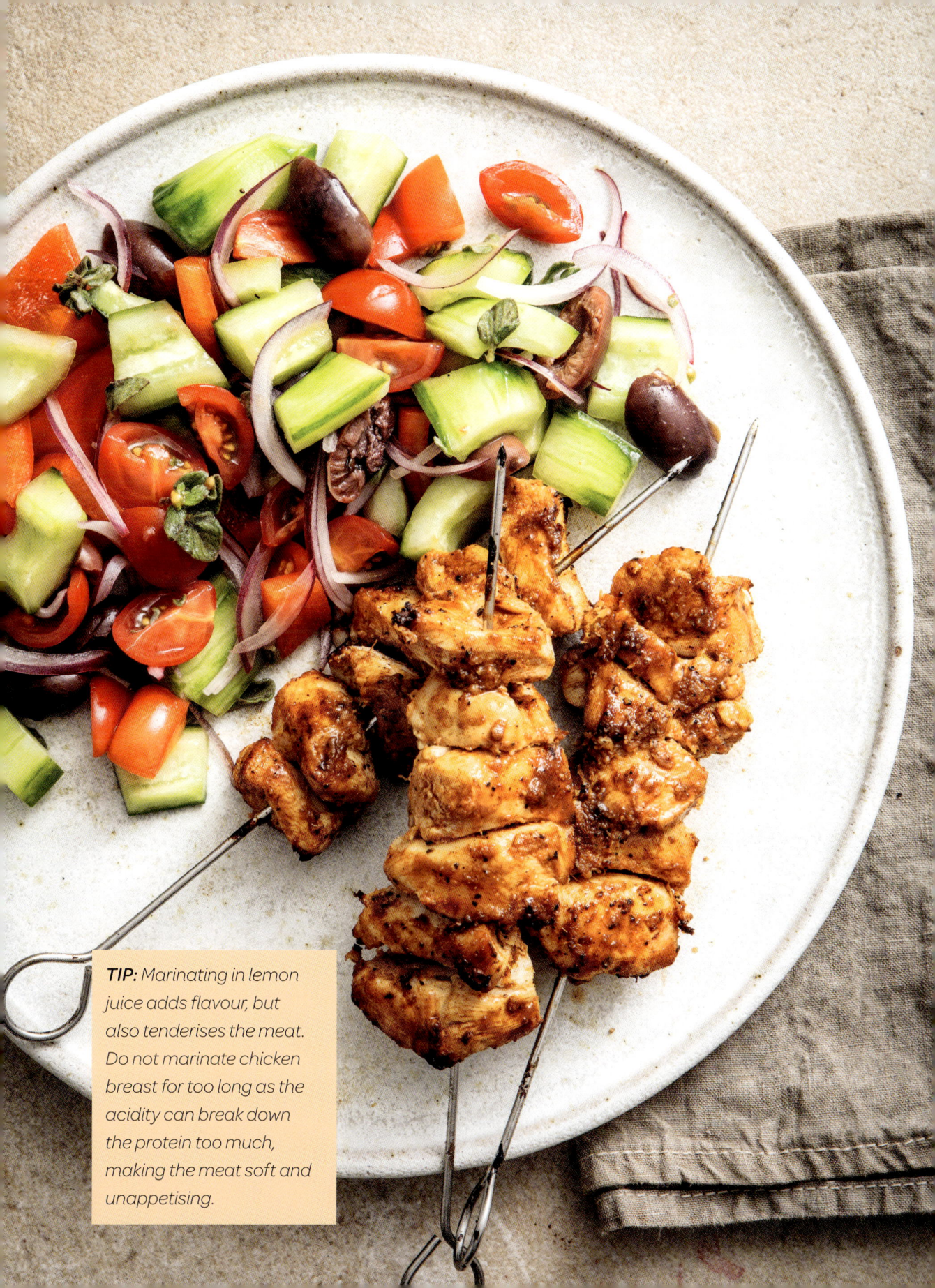

TIP: *Marinating in lemon juice adds flavour, but also tenderises the meat. Do not marinate chicken breast for too long as the acidity can break down the protein too much, making the meat soft and unappetising.*

CHILLI BEEF TACOS

Who doesn't love a taco? These cool and crunchy baby gem leaves make excellent wraps for the warm, smoky, garlicky beef mince. This recipe is a truly glorious combination of flavours and a perfect mid-week supper. For a family and friends version serve with guacamole, cheese and corn tacos. The mince is great for batch cooking and freezes well.

SERVES 2
PREP: 10 MINUTES
COOK: 30 MINUTES

60g onion, finely diced
50g carrot, finely diced
35g celery, finely diced
450ml chicken or vegetable stock
260g minced beef
15g/1 tbsp tomato purée*
2 large garlic cloves, crushed
2 tsp smoked paprika*
½ tsp chilli powder*
100g baby gem lettuce leaves, whole
sliced fresh mild chilli* and chopped fresh coriander, to serve (optional)
sea salt and freshly ground black pepper

1. Cook the onion, carrot and celery with a pinch of salt in a splash of stock to soften for about 5 minutes.
2. Add the mince and cook until brown, then add the tomato purée, garlic, smoked paprika, chilli and the remaining stock.
3. Simmer gently for 20–30 minutes until the stock has reduced to become a syrupy, spicy coating for the cooked mince.
4. Check the seasoning, adding salt and pepper if necessary.
5. Pile the warm spicy beef into the baby gem leaves and scatter with fresh sliced chilli and coriander.

VARIATION
- If you are avoiding nightshades, replace the tomato purée with additional carrot and omit the chilli powder and paprika.

BOLOGNESE

A delicious go-to mince recipe; serve with spiralised butternut squash for our take on spaghetti Bolognese. I've chosen spiralised squash as it holds its shape and adds a sweet note, but the mince is also delicious served with courgetti. The deeply savoury mince is a suppertime staple; I always have a batch in the freezer – it's so useful when you are low on time and have a family to feed.

SERVES 2
PREP: 10 MINUTES
COOK: 25 MINUTES

260g lean minced beef
400ml fresh chicken or vegetable stock
10g/2 tsp tomato purée* (optional)
50g onion, finely diced
30g carrot, finely diced
20g celery, finely diced
3 garlic cloves, finely chopped
2 sprigs of fresh thyme
1 bay leaf
150g butternut squash, peeled and spiralised
sea salt and freshly ground black pepper

1. In a saucepan, cook the mince with a splash of stock until it browns. Add the tomato purée and cook for a minute more.
2. Add the onion, carrot, celery, garlic, the remaining stock, thyme and bay leaf and season with salt and pepper. Simmer over a low heat for about 20 minutes until the stock has reduced to a syrupy gravy.
3. Remove the bay leaf and thyme, taste and season with salt and pepper.
4. Cook the squash in salted boiling water for 2–3 minutes, drain and serve immediately with the mince.

VARIATION
- If you are avoiding nightshades, replace the tomato purée with 10g of extra carrot.

TIP: For a friends and family version, serve with wholewheat pasta and cheese.

SCANDI MACKEREL SALAD

This is my number one go-to lunch; I have it at least twice a week! The flavour combination of salty oily fish, sweet fridge-cold apples, fiery mustard and fragrant dill is a Scandinavian classic. Cucumber, radish and chicory add a cool, peppery crunch. Adding apple to the salad makes it enormous and leaves you feeling as though you've had a very satisfying and substantial meal. I've used smoked mackerel, but you could use fresh or tinned salmon or trout.

SERVES 2
PREP: 10 MINUTES

FOR THE MUSTARD DRESSING
1 tbsp apple cider vinegar
1 tsp Colman's mustard powder
splash of cold water
sea salt and freshly ground black pepper

FOR THE MACKEREL
140g chicory, roughly chopped
80g cucumber, finely sliced
2 fridge-cold apples, finely sliced into matchsticks
40g radishes, finely sliced
2 tbsp roughly chopped fresh dill
260g smoked mackerel fillets

1. To make the dressing, whisk the apple cider vinegar, mustard powder, salt and pepper and a splash of cold water together in a large serving bowl.
2. Add the chicory, cucumber, apple, radish and dill, then toss to evenly dress the salad. Flake the fish over the top. Eat immediately.

> **VARIATIONS**
> - The mild aniseed flavour of dill is not to everyone's taste, so feel free to replace it with chives.
> - The chicory can be replaced with salad leaves.
> - However, the apple, fish and mustard are what make this salad unmistakably Scandinavian and are therefore non-negotiable!

> **TIP:** *Making the dressing in your serving dish saves on waste and washing up!*

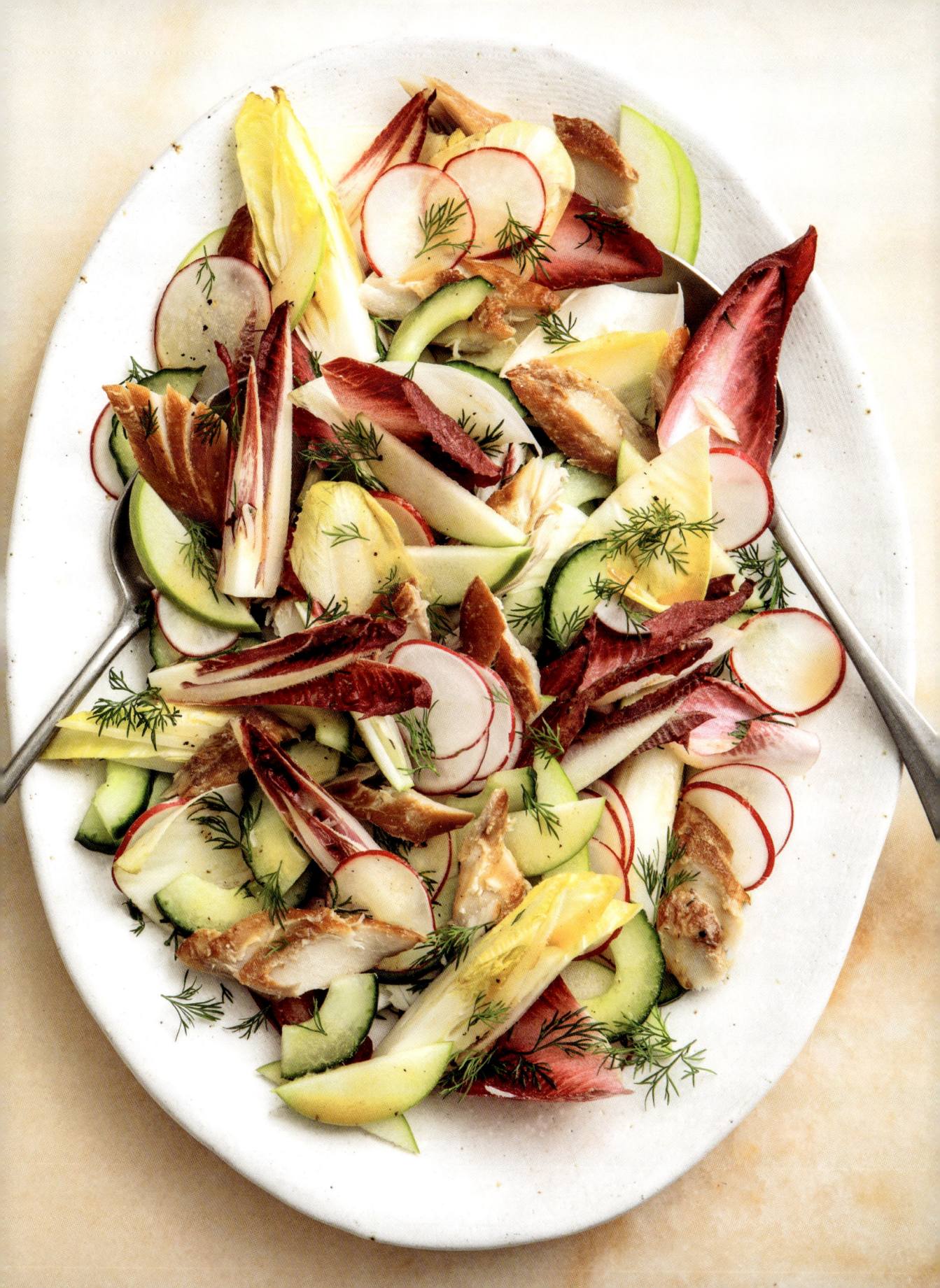

Comfort

BRAISED CHICKEN WITH FONDANT LEEKS & FENNEL

This is proper comfort food; a bowl of steaming deliciousness. Fennel and leeks become silky and unctuous when braised in umami-rich broth. Woody thyme and fragrant garlic marry perfectly with succulent, poached chicken to complete the dish. It's a simple, savoury meal that really does feel like a hug in a bowl.

SERVES 2
PREP: 10 MINUTES
COOK: 1 HOUR

350ml fresh chicken stock
130g fennel bulb, cut into 2cm wedges
130g leeks, halved lengthways and sliced into 3cm pieces
3 garlic cloves, thinly sliced
3–4 sprigs of fresh thyme
260g chicken breasts
chopped fresh parsley and a squeeze of fresh lemon juice, to serve (optional)
sea salt and freshly ground black pepper

1. Preheat the oven to 180°C/160°C fan/gas mark 4.
2. Warm a generous splash of stock in a shallow ovenproof pan with a lid and add the fennel, leeks and a grind of salt and pepper.
3. Cook over a medium heat for about 5–10 minutes until the vegetables begin to caramelise and soften.
4. Add the remaining stock, garlic and thyme, cover tightly with a lid and transfer to the oven for 15 minutes.
5. Remove the lid and nestle the chicken breasts among the vegetables. Cover and return to the oven for a further 20–25 minutes until the chicken is cooked and opaque.
6. Remove the chicken pieces and keep them warm, then return the vegetables to the oven to cook uncovered for a final 10 minutes. This will allow the stock to reduce and the vegetables to caramelise slightly and intensify in flavour.
7. Serve in a bowl with a generous grind of black pepper, a squeeze of lemon juice and a scattering of fresh parsley.

TIP: *To prepare the fennel wedges, keep the base intact so the layers hold together.*

CLASSIC BEEF STEW WITH THYME

I've used my beef stew and dumplings recipe for decades, and it's a family favourite. When I discovered HBD, I ditched the dumplings but looked for a way of keeping the flavours of my original stew. This is the result. Fresh thyme and tender beef in a dark gravy, sweetened with carrots and with the umami depth of tamari. It has been given a big thumbs up by the whole family. Scale this up, as it's brilliant to have some in the freezer for dark, wintry evenings.

SERVES 2
PREP: 10 MINUTES
COOK: 2½ HOURS

260g stewing or braising steak, cut into pieces
100ml water, freshly boiled
60g onion, sliced
2 garlic cloves, finely chopped
90g carrot, roughly chopped
2 tsp (10g) tomato purée*
1½ tbsp tamari
250ml fresh chicken stock
4–5 sprigs of fresh thyme
1 bay leaf
100g cabbage, sliced
sea salt and freshly ground black pepper

> **VARIATION**
> - If you are avoiding nightshades, replace the tomato purée with an extra 10g of carrot or onion.

1. Preheat the oven to 170°C/150°C fan/gas mark 3.
2. Season the beef with salt and pepper. Seal in a non-stick frying pan over a medium–high heat. Turn the meat regularly to ensure it is burnished and browned on all sides. Transfer to a casserole dish.
3. Deglaze the frying pan with the boiling water, scraping up all the meat juices and sticky residues. This will add colour and depth of flavour.
4. Add the onion to the frying pan and cook gently for 2–3 minutes until golden. Add the garlic and continue to cook for a further minute. Transfer the mixture to the casserole dish.
5. Finally, add the carrot, tomato purée, tamari, stock, thyme and bay leaf to the casserole and season with a good grind of black pepper.
6. Cover tightly with foil or a lid and cook in the oven for 2½ hours until the meat is meltingly tender.
7. Remove the meat and vegetables from the casserole dish with a slotted spoon and keep warm. Pour the cooking liquid into a saucepan. Boil continuously until the liquid has reduced by two-thirds and becomes dark and a little syrupy. This takes about 5–10 minutes for these quantities, but longer if you are cooking a larger quantity.
8. While the sauce is reducing, cook the cabbage in a little water with a grind of salt and pepper for about 5 minutes until it wilts and softens.
9. Pour the gravy over the beef and vegetables and serve.

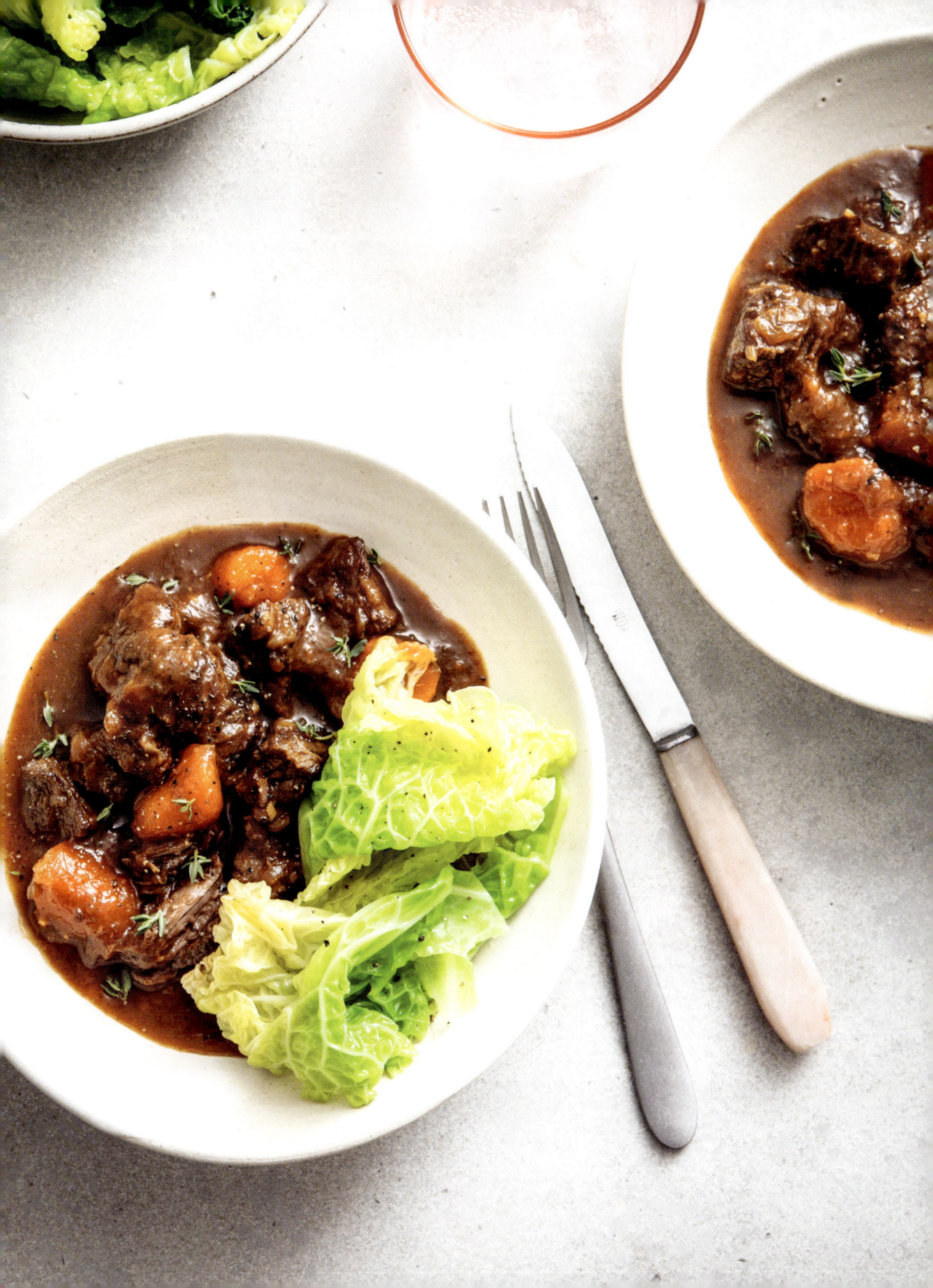

ITALIAN PORK & FENNEL MEATBALLS

This recipe is inspired by the fabulous meatballs served at our favourite Italian restaurant, fragrant with fennel and chilli and poached in a gloriously rich sauce to ensure they stay succulent and juicy. You can use roasted red peppers from a jar, or make your own. The meatballs freeze well and are great for batch cooking.

SERVES 2
PREP: 10 MINUTES
COOK: 25 MINUTES

FOR THE MEATBALLS
260g lean pork mince
3 garlic cloves, crushed
2 tbsp finely chopped fresh parsley
½ tsp fennel seeds
½ tsp chilli flakes* (optional)
sea salt and freshly ground black pepper

FOR THE SAUCE
150g red peppers*, deseeded and quartered
20g onion, finely chopped
1 garlic clove, crushed
20g/4 tsp tomato purée*
250ml water, freshly boiled
70g courgette, very thinly sliced
chopped fresh parsley, to serve
sea salt and freshly ground black pepper

1. Make the meatballs by combining the minced pork, garlic, parsley, fennel seeds and chilli flakes (if using) in a bowl. Mix well and season generously with salt and pepper. Use your hands to shape the mixture into 12 meatballs.
2. Preheat the oven to 200°C/180°C fan/gas mark 6.
3. To make the sauce, roast the red pepper pieces for about 35 minutes until they are soft. Purée in a blender until smooth.
4. In a non-stick pan with a lid, cook the onion in a splash of cold water over a medium heat for about 3–4 minutes until soft. Add the garlic, tomato purée, red pepper purée, boiling water and a grind of salt and pepper to make a sauce.
5. Drop the meatballs into the sauce, cover the pan with a lid and simmer over a low heat for 15 minutes, turning over the meatballs regularly.
6. Add the courgette and continue to cook for a further 5 minutes uncovered, until the sauce has reduced and thickened and the courgette has softened.
7. Check the meatballs are cooked through and serve sprinkled with fresh parsley.

VARIATION
- If you are avoiding nightshades, you can have the meatballs without the sauce. Omit the chilli flakes and bake the meatballs covered with foil for 15–20 minutes. Serve with steamed vegetables or spiralised courgetti.

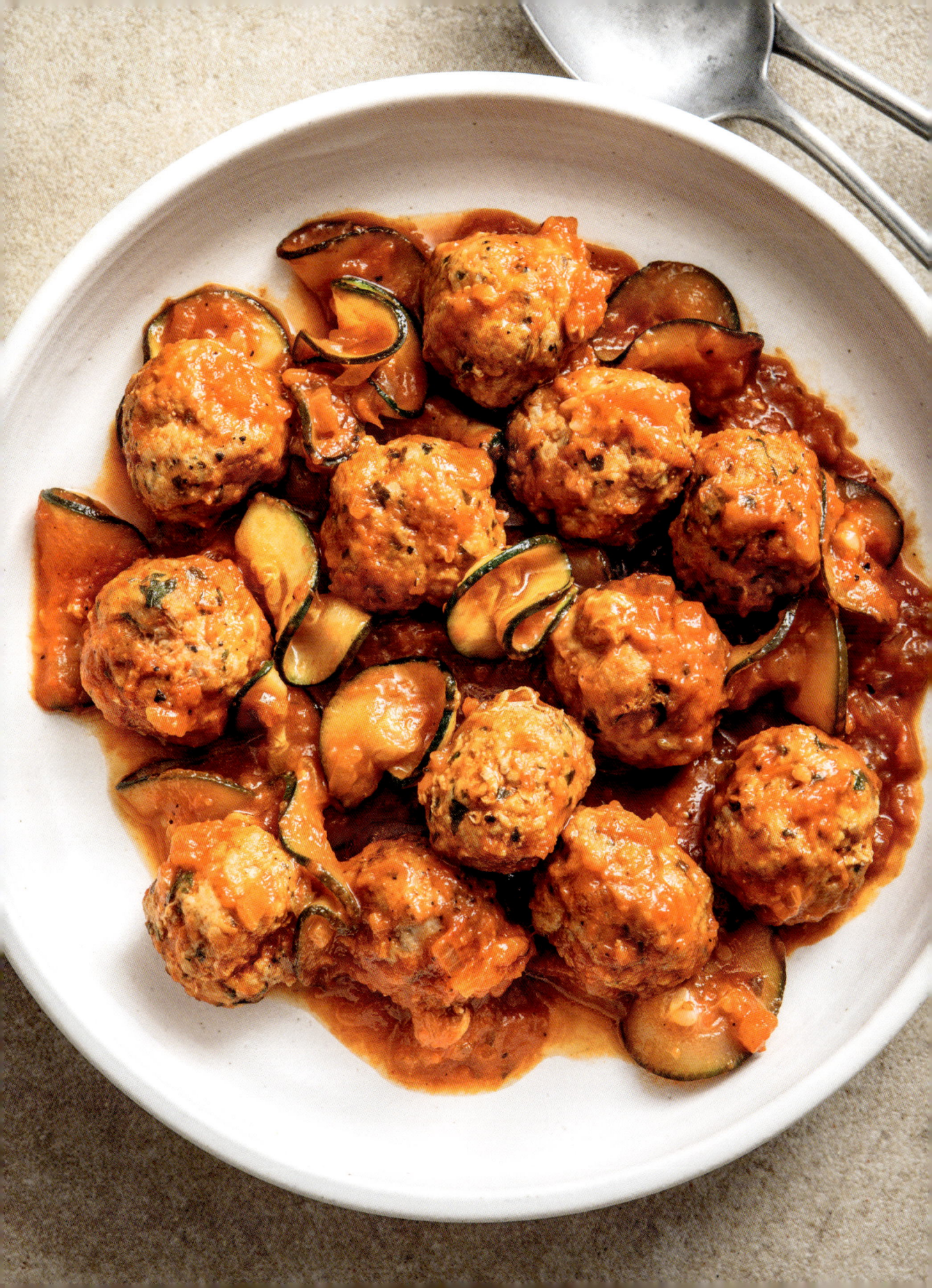

STEAMING HUNGARIAN MEATBALL BROTH

This dish was dreamt up on a bitterly cold January day. It's a substantial, deeply savoury broth, which takes on the flavour of the fragrant meatballs and vegetables. A real crowd pleaser, this is the perfect recipe to scale up for a crowd, making it a truly nourishing and comforting winter warmer. This dish freezes well and is perfect for batch cooking.

SERVES 2
PREP: 15 MINUTES
COOK: 25 MINUTES

- 4 tbsp chopped fresh parsley
- 2 garlic cloves, crushed
- 260g pork mince
- 60g onion, finely chopped
- 500ml fresh chicken or vegetable stock
- 60g carrots, roughly chopped
- 60g celery, roughly chopped
- 80g green cabbage, roughly chopped
- sea salt and freshly ground black pepper

1. First make the meatballs. Mix 2 tablespoons of the parsley and the garlic with the mince, season generously with salt and pepper and shape into small balls. Put in the fridge to firm up.
2. Make the broth. In a saucepan, cook the onion in a little of the stock for 5 minutes to soften. Add the remaining stock, carrots and celery and simmer over a low heat for a further 5 minutes.
3. Carefully drop the meatballs into the hot broth, cover the pan with a lid and continue to simmer over a low heat for 15–20 minutes until the meatballs are cooked. Add the cabbage and cook with the lid on for a further few minutes until the cabbage is soft and wilted.
4. Serve in a soup bowl sprinkled with the remaining parsley and a generous grind of black pepper.

BUTTERNUT & SAGE RISOTTO

Sweet butternut squash and woody sage are a classic partnership in Italian cookery. This dish is filling and comforting, ideal for a lunchtime when you know you have a busy afternoon ahead and need extra energy. I highly recommend the chickpea rice by Mr Organic, which has a firm bite and tastes a little like orzo pasta. This dish freezes well.

SERVES 2
PREP: 10 MINUTES
COOK: 20–25 MINUTES

60g shallot or onion, finely diced
300ml chicken or vegetable stock
160g butternut squash, peeled and finely diced
3 garlic cloves, finely sliced
160g chickpea rice
250ml boiling water
40g baby spinach leaves
2 tsp finely chopped fresh sage
sea salt and freshly ground black pepper

1. In a shallow non-stick pan, gently cook the shallot in a splash of stock for 3–4 minutes over a low heat.
2. Add the butternut squash and garlic, and cook for a further minute before adding the rice, the rest of the stock, the boiling water and a generous pinch of salt and pepper.
3. Increase the heat slightly and cook for 15 minutes, stirring occasionally.
4. Add the spinach and sage and cook for 2 minutes until the spinach has wilted. Most of the liquid will have evaporated, but if it hasn't, turn up the heat a little and cook for a further minute.
5. Test that the rice is cooked; it should be al dente.
6. Season with a generous grind of black pepper and a pinch of sea salt if necessary.

MOROCCAN LAMB CASSEROLE WITH SQUASH & SPINACH

With gentle fragrant spicing, sweet butternut squash and lamb so tender it falls apart; this tagine is a true one-pot wonder. So easy to make – it's a satisfying, nourishing and comforting meal. We eat this family favourite regularly with a side dish of couscous and a scattering of toasted, flaked almonds for the kids. It's perfect for batch cooking and you can use beef instead of lamb if you prefer.

SERVES 2
PREP: 10 MINUTES
COOK: 2 HOURS 15 MINUTES

260g boned lamb neck, cut into 2–3cm pieces
300ml fresh chicken or vegetable stock
3 garlic cloves, sliced
40g onion, finely chopped
20g/4 tsp tomato purée*
1 tsp ras el hanout
½ tsp ground cumin
160g butternut squash, peeled, seeds removed and flesh cut into 2–3cm pieces
40g baby spinach
sea salt and freshly ground black pepper

1. Preheat the oven to 160°C/140°C fan/gas mark 3.
2. Seal the lamb pieces by frying in a dry non-stick pan over a medium–high heat. Cook for about 4–5 minutes, turning regularly until all sides are slightly burnished and nicely browned. This caramelisation creates the deep flavour and colour. Transfer the lamb to an ovenproof dish.
3. Add the stock to briefly deglaze the frying pan, scraping up any sticky meat juices. Add the garlic, onion, tomato purée, ras el hanout and cumin. Simmer for 1–2 minutes to combine all the flavours. Pour over the lamb, seal tightly with foil and transfer to the oven for 1¾ hours.
4. Remove the dish from the oven and turn up the heat to 190°C/170°C fan/gas mark 5.
5. Remove the foil and add the squash pieces to the lamb, stir and return the dish to the oven. Cook uncovered for about 25 minutes until the squash has softened.
6. Finally, add the spinach and a generous grind of salt and pepper, stir well and return to the oven. Cook for a further 5 minutes or until the spinach has wilted into the sauce.

> **VARIATION**
> - If you are avoiding nightshades, replace the tomato purée with 20g of sliced mushrooms.

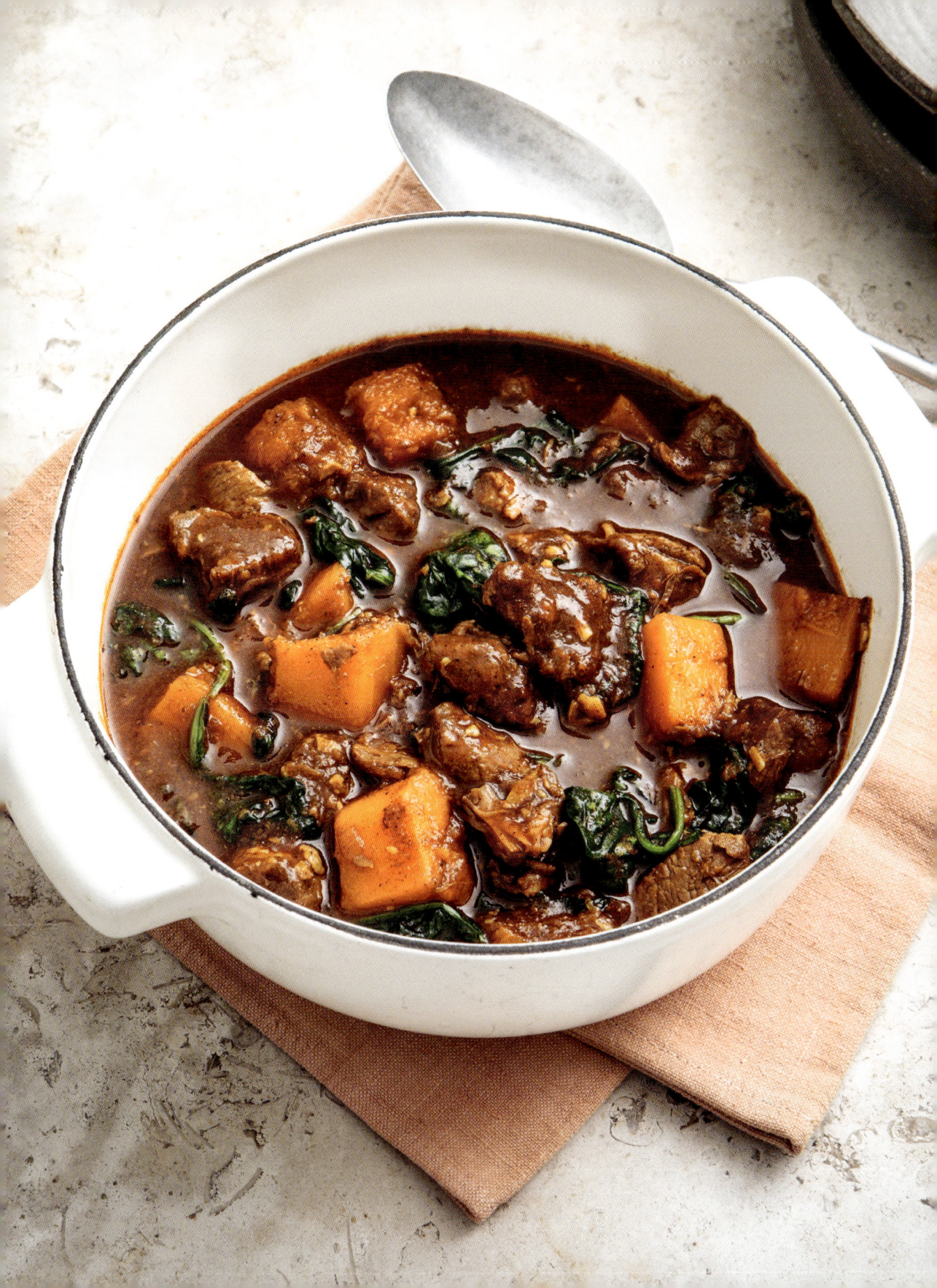

PISTOU SOUP WITH PARMESAN CRISPS

In this traditional Provençal dish the simple ingredients combine to create a delicate vegetable soup. The classic French flavours of basil and garlic – with a hint of aniseed, courtesy of the fennel – elevate the vegetables, while the Parmesan adds rich umami flavour. Dicing all the vegetables to the same size is key so that they cook evenly and give the soup a pared-back elegance. This is another example of a dish in which the whole is greater than the sum of its parts. I serve this soup regularly to friends who are, without exception, suitably impressed. The dazzling green of the soup and delicate Parmesan crisps look beautiful and inviting.

SERVES 2
PREP: 15 MINUTES
COOK: 20 MINUTES

30g onion, finely diced
30g carrot, finely diced
30g celery, finely diced
40g fennel, finely diced
400ml boiling water
60g courgette, finely diced
20g cherry tomatoes*
50g green beans, finely sliced
1 tbsp Pistou (see page 58)
20g Parmesan, grated, to serve
sea salt and freshly ground white pepper

FOR THE PARMESAN CRISPS
140g Parmesan, grated

1. Preheat the oven to 230°C/210°C fan/gas mark 8.
2. First make the Parmesan crisps. Place 8 separate mounds of grated Parmesan on a non-stick baking sheet. Leave a little space around each mound, as they will spread as they melt.
3. Cook for 7–8 minutes until the cheese has melted and is dark golden at its edges.
4. Remove from the oven and leave to cool completely.
5. To make the soup, put the onion, carrot, celery and fennel into a saucepan with a splash of the boiling water. Season with a pinch of salt and white pepper. Simmer gently for 5–6 minutes to soften the vegetables.
6. Add the remaining boiling water, courgette, tomatoes and the green beans. Continue to simmer for about 4–5 minutes, by which time the vegetables will be soft but still retain some bite.
7. Remove from the heat, stir in the pistou and check the seasoning, adding more salt, white pepper or pistou to taste.
8. Sprinkle with Parmesan and serve the Parmesan crisps alongside.

VARIATION
- If you are avoiding nightshades, replace the cherry tomatoes with an additional 20g of carrot or celery.

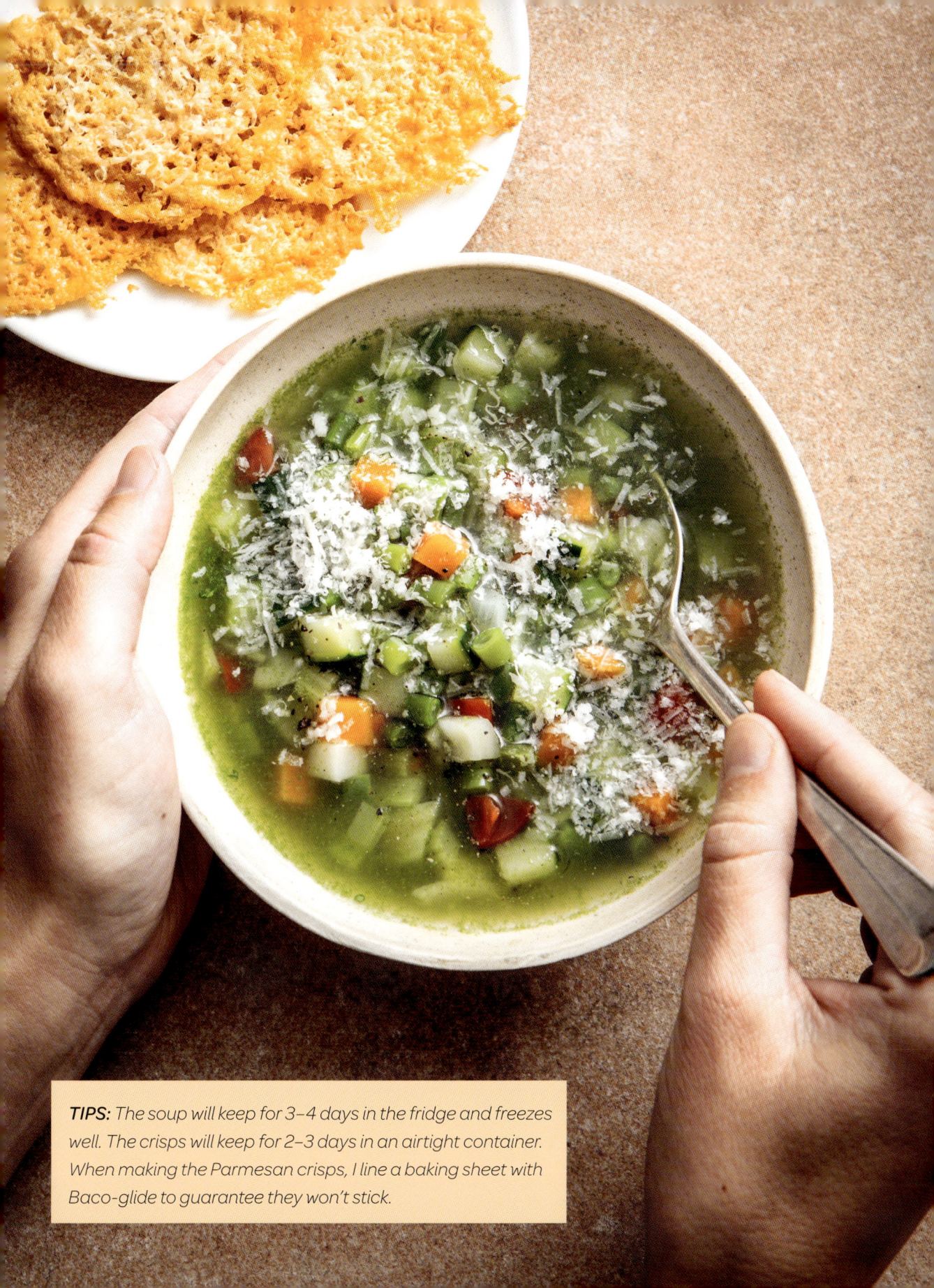

TIPS: *The soup will keep for 3–4 days in the fridge and freezes well. The crisps will keep for 2–3 days in an airtight container. When making the Parmesan crisps, I line a baking sheet with Baco-glide to guarantee they won't stick.*

SMOKY VEGGIE GOULASH

In this version of Hungary's national dish, sweet butternut squash and peppers balance the rich, peppery sauce. The addition of whole butter beans makes this a hearty main course, while puréed butter beans with lemon juice and garlic are a fabulous substitute for sour cream. This dish freezes well.

SERVES 2
PREP: 10 MINUTES
COOK: 25 MINUTES

40g red onion, finely chopped
250ml chicken or vegetable stock
3 garlic cloves, finely chopped
60g red pepper*, roughly chopped
2 tsp paprika*
a pinch of cayenne pepper*
150g butternut squash, peeled and roughly chopped
10g/2tsp tomato purée*
240g cooked butter beans
chopped fresh parsley and chives, to serve
sea salt and freshly ground black pepper

FOR THE BUTTER BEAN CREAM
80g cooked butter beans
1 small garlic clove, crushed
a squeeze of lemon juice
a splash of cold water

1. Prepare the goulash. In a saucepan over a medium heat, cook the onion in a splash of stock for about 4–5 minutes until soft.
2. Add the garlic, red pepper, paprika and cayenne and cook for a further minute before adding the butternut squash, the rest of the stock, tomato purée and some salt and pepper. Cover with a lid and simmer for about 15 minutes.
3. Add the butter beans and continue to simmer uncovered for about 10 minutes until the butternut squash is tender. Top up with a little boiling water if necessary.
4. Meanwhile, make the butter bean cream. Purée the butter beans, garlic, lemon juice and a grind of salt and pepper. Add splashes of cold water until the purée is the consistency of double cream and silky smooth.
5. Serve the goulash topped with a swirl of butter bean cream and a sprinkling of fresh parsley or chives.

TEMPEH CHILLI WITH CAULIFLOWER RICE

Tempeh mince, made from fermented soy, is crumbly and savoury, making it perfect for this robust, rich and smoky chilli. Tempeh is a staple of Indonesian cookery. It is high in fibre, protein and nutrients and your gut microbes will love it! This dish freezes well. This recipe is not suitable for those avoiding nightshades.

SERVES 2
PREP: 10 MINUTES
COOK: 30 MINUTES

40g red onion, finely diced
300ml vegetable stock
2 garlic cloves, crushed
20g celery, finely diced
30g carrot, finely diced
50g red pepper*, finely sliced
2 tsp smoked paprika*
½ tsp chilli flakes*
½ tsp ground cumin
260g organic tempeh mince
20g/4 tsp tomato purée*
100g cauliflower rice
   (see page 140)
fresh parsley, to serve
sea salt and freshly ground
   black pepper

1. In a medium-sized pan, cook the onion in a splash of stock over a medium heat for 4–5 minutes to soften.
2. Add the garlic, celery, carrot and red pepper and cook for a further 2–3 minutes.
3. Add the smoked paprika, chilli flakes, cumin, tempeh, the rest of the stock and the tomato purée. Partially cover with a lid and simmer gently for 15–20 minutes. Remove the lid and continue simmering, stirring occasionally, for a further 10 minutes.
4. Meanwhile, in a small pan, cook the cauliflower rice in a splash of water for 5 minutes until tender.
5. Check the seasoning, add salt and pepper if necessary and serve scattered with fresh parsley.

CHANA MASALA WITH FLATBREADS

A gently fragrant vegan curry with a rich sweet gravy, thanks to the addition of butternut squash. Adding fresh onion to the curry paste and mincing it along with the spices creates the basis for a slightly thicker sauce, perfect for mopping up with the gorgeous little flatbreads. This curry is seriously filling, comforting and, most importantly, delicious! Both the chana masala and the flatbreads freeze well. It's delicious served with Mango Chutney (see page 61).

SERVES 2
PREP: 10 MINUTES
COOK: 25 MINUTES

80g onion, chopped
3 garlic cloves, sliced
2 tsp ground coriander
2 tsp mild curry powder
1 tsp ground cumin
½ tsp ground ginger
250ml vegetable stock
60g butternut squash, peeled and finely diced
40g tomato*, finely diced
160g chickpeas, cooked
80g baby spinach
fresh coriander, to serve
sea salt and freshly ground black pepper

FOR THE FLATBREADS
80g chickpea (gram) flour
130ml cold water

1. Put the onion, garlic, coriander, curry powder, cumin, ginger and a splash of stock in a blender. Pulse briefly to create a loose paste.
2. Put the paste in a pan and simmer for about 2–3 minutes before adding the butternut squash, tomato, a pinch of salt and pepper and the remaining stock.
3. Cover with a lid and simmer for 10 minutes.
4. Make the batter for the flatbreads by whisking the chickpea flour, water and salt. Leave to rest.
5. Add the chickpeas to the chana masala and continue to cook uncovered for 5 minutes until the butternut is soft.
6. Add the spinach and cook for a final few minutes until it has wilted.
7. Check the seasoning and add more salt and pepper if necessary. Keep warm while you make the flatbreads.
8. Heat a non-stick frying pan over a medium heat and carefully drop a tablespoon of the batter into the pan. After 1–2 minutes small bubbles will appear on the surface of the flatbread. Flip it over and cook for a further minute or 2 until it is spongy and slightly golden at the edges. Repeat until you have used all the batter.
9. Serve the chana masala sprinkled with fresh coriander and the breads piled alongside.

> **VARIATION**
> - If you are avoiding nightshades, you can replace the tomato with additional butternut squash.

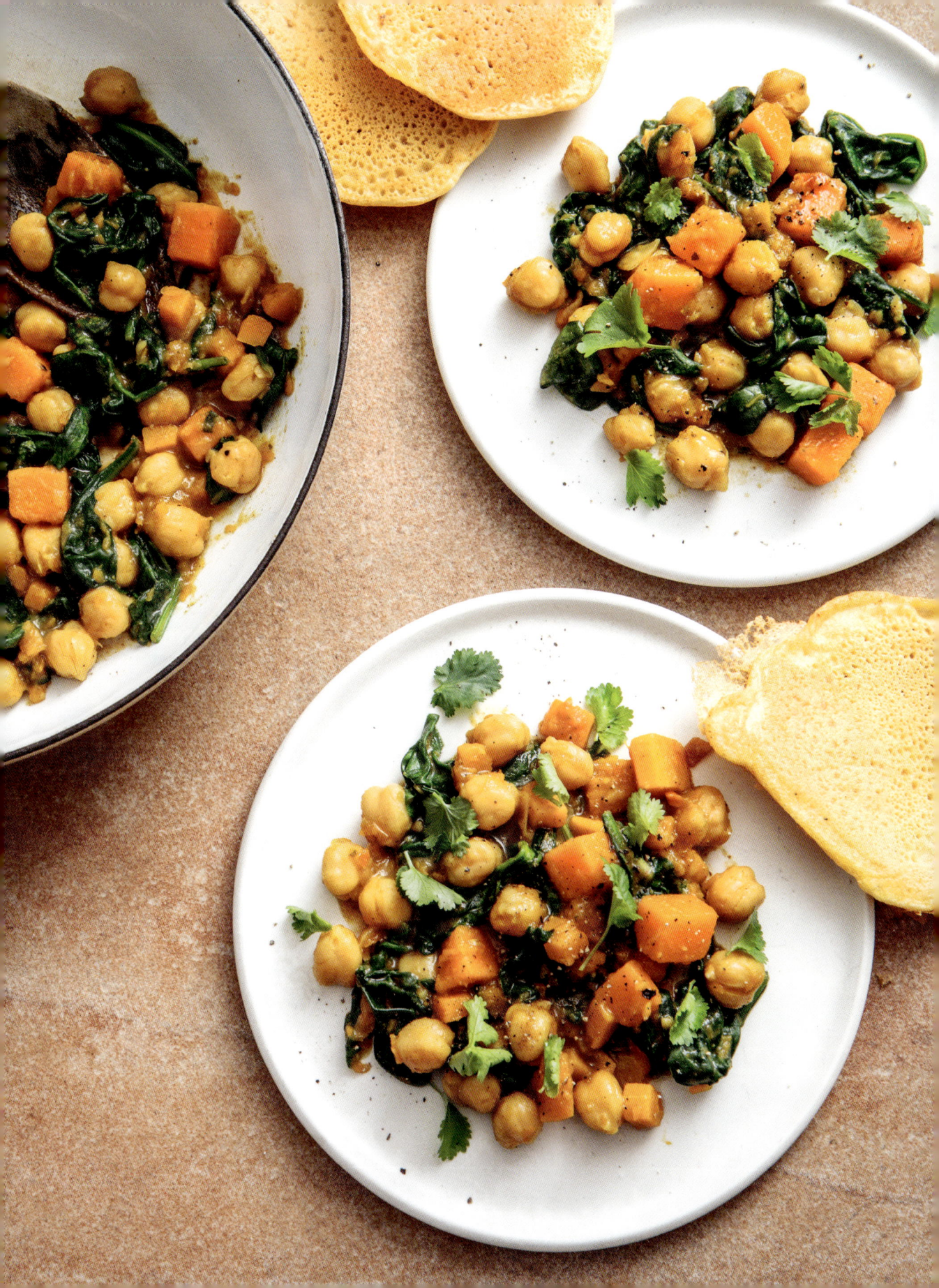

Simple, Speedy Suppers

BAKED SEA BREAM WITH MASH & GREENS

Sometimes we really don't need all the bells and whistles: simple and comforting food is the order of the day. This dish was inspired by a lunch in Paris decades ago of Dover sole and *pommes purée*. I still remember the joy of it, the creamy, slightly peppery mash with the firm, flaky white fish. It was ridiculously good and deeply comforting.

SERVES 2
PREP: 10 MINUTES
COOK: 40 MINUTES

200g cauliflower florets
260g sea bream fillets
60g spring greens, chopped
sea salt and freshly ground white pepper

1. Preheat the oven to 190°C/170°C fan/gas mark 5.
2. Parcel up the cauliflower florets in foil with a splash of water. Bake for 35–45 minutes until very soft.
3. Season the sea bream fillets with salt and pepper. Bake in the oven for 15 minutes.
4. Remove the cauliflower from the oven. Carefully unwrap the florets and put in a food processor along with the residual cooking liquid. Season with a pinch of salt and white pepper. Purée until silky smooth.
5. Briefly cook the spring greens in a splash of water and season with salt and pepper.
6. Carefully remove the fish from the oven and peel off the skin.
7. Serve the fish on a bed of cauliflower mash with the greens alongside.

LEMON & ROSEMARY MONKFISH SKEWERS

Monkfish is deliciously sweet and firm – and robust enough to absorb a sharp, zingy citrus marinade before being gently steamed. Courgettes, tender and fresh, are gorgeous alongside the fish and fragrant rosemary. Serve with a simple salad of dressed leaves sprinkled with apple cider vinegar and sea salt. The skewers are also glorious with a few spoonfuls of sweet and smoky pepper ketchup.

SERVES 2
PREP: 15 MINUTES
COOK: 12 MINUTES

zest and juice of 1 lemon,
1 tbsp finely chopped fresh rosemary
260g monkfish, cut into 2–3cm cubes
200g courgette, cut into slices
60g salad leaves, to serve
sea salt and freshly ground black pepper

1. Combine the lemon zest and juice and the rosemary with a pinch of salt and a good grind of black pepper. Add the monkfish, mix well to coat and set aside for 10 minutes to marinate.
2. Set a large pan of water to the boil and line the base of a steamer with parchment paper.
3. Assemble the skewers by alternating courgette slices with the monkfish cubes.
4. Once the water is boiling, steam the skewers for about 12 minutes until the fish is opaque and cooked through.

VARIATION
- Swap the salad laves for 4 tbsp Red Pepper Ketchup (see page 56).

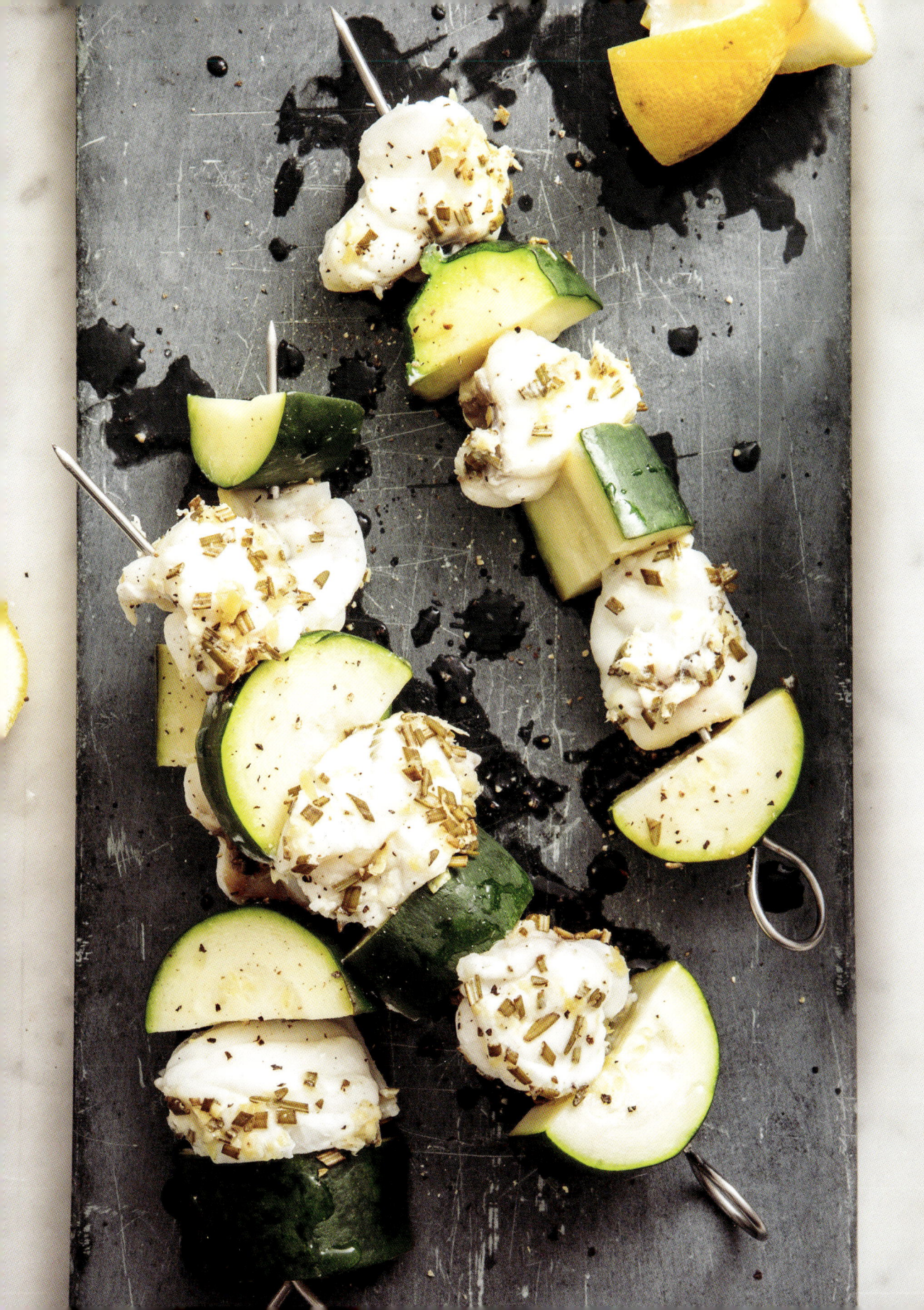

AROMATIC BAKED BASS EN PAPILLOTE

I love to cook fish the French way, *en papillote*, which literally translates as 'in paper'. The parchment paper parcel creates steam, so there is no need for oil. This recipe is super easy to prepare in advance and pop in the oven. Sea bass is a robust, oily fish full of flavour, and used a lot in Chinese cookery. It works brilliantly with ginger and can hold its own with fragrant Asian flavours.

SERVES 2
PREP: 10 MINUTES (PLUS 15 MINUTES MARINADING)
COOK: 20 MINUTES

3 tbsp tamari
2 garlic cloves, crushed
5cm piece fresh ginger, peeled and finely julienned
2 tbsp finely chopped fresh coriander stalks
260g sea bass or bream fillets
140g pak choi, roughly chopped lengthways
40g carrot, finely julienned
30g leek, finely julienned
30g courgette, julienned
20g spring onion, julienned
chopped fresh coriander leaves, to serve

1. Preheat the oven to 180°C/160°C fan/gas mark 4.
2. To make the marinade, mix the tamari, garlic, ginger and coriander stalks. Use a sharp knife to make 4 or 5 shallow slashes in the skin of the bass to allow the marinade to penetrate. Coat the fish with the marinade and set aside for 10–15 minutes.
3. Divide the pak choi, carrot, leek, courgette and spring onion into two piles. Take two pieces of parchment paper and pile the vegetables in the centre of each piece to create a bed for the fish.
4. Lay the marinated fish on the vegetables, making sure to pour over any residual marinade in the dish. Add 2–3 tablespoons cold water and wrap both parcels loosely, ensuring they are sealed to trap the steam.
5. Bake for 20 minutes. The fish will be perfectly cooked and the vegetables al dente.
6. Remove the skin from the fish (optional), scatter with the coriander and serve in the parcel so you don't lose any of the delicious cooking juices.

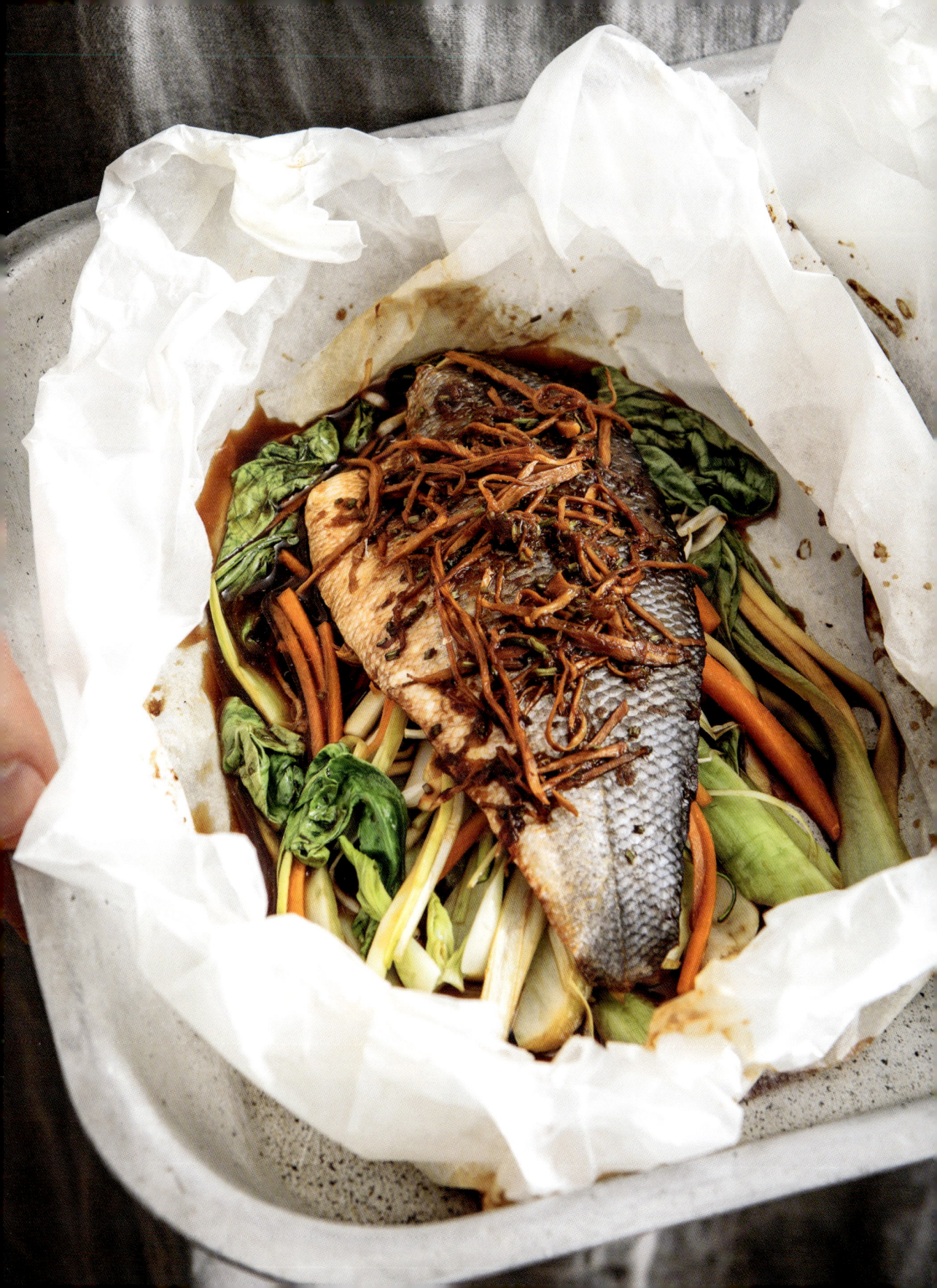

CHICKEN CAULIFLOWER RICE PILAF

This quick and easy chicken pilaf is savoury and satisfying; a perfect warming meal made with store cupboard and freezer staples. The cauliflower rice absorbs the subtle flavours of chicken, vegetables and herbs; a squeeze of lemon before serving adds a fresh note that really brings the flavours to life. Sofrito is a combination of finely diced onion, celery and carrot – it's available in many supermarkets, already prepared and frozen in bags.

SERVES 2
PREP: 10 MINUTES
COOK: 20 MINUTES

40g onion, finely diced
40g celery, finely diced
40g carrot, finely diced
250ml fresh chicken or vegetable stock
2 large garlic cloves, finely sliced
260g chicken breast, finely diced
1 bay leaf
140g cauliflower rice (see page 140)
1–2 tbsp chopped fresh flat-leaf parsley
squeeze of lemon, to serve (optional)
sea salt and freshly ground black pepper

1. In a non-stick pan, cook the onion, celery and carrot in a splash of stock for about 5 minutes until soft.
2. Add the garlic, chicken, bay leaf and the remaining stock. Gently simmer for about 10 minutes to allow the chicken to cook and the stock to reduce.
3. Add the cauliflower rice and continue to cook with the lid off for about 5 minutes until all the liquid has evaporated.
4. Take the pan off the heat, remove the bay leaf and add the parsley, a generous pinch of salt and pepper and a squeeze of lemon to serve.

TRUFFLE MUSHROOM TARTS WITH EMMENTAL

This dish is inspired by my old favourite, the Ole & Steen truffle mushroom focaccia. Oodles of gooey cheese, crispy and slightly scorched around the edges, on a base of umami-rich mushrooms, fragrant woody thyme and earthy spinach. A real treat for the taste buds when seasoned with indulgent truffle salt. The peppery rocket garnish, sprinkled with zingy apple cider vinegar, balances the rich flavours of the cheese and truffle perfectly.

SERVES 2
PREP: 10 MINUTES
COOK: 10 MINUTES

190g portobello mushrooms, very finely sliced
160g Emmental cheese, sliced or grated
40g baby spinach
1 tsp fresh thyme leaves
a pinch of truffle salt (optional)
30g rocket leaves
1 tsp apple cider vinegar
sea salt and freshly ground black pepper

TIPS: *We use Truffle Hunter truffle salt. Use a mandolin or very sharp knife to slice the mushrooms into wafer-thin strips.*

1. Preheat the grill to medium.
2. On a non-stick baking tray, use the mushroom strips to make two circular discs about 12–15cm in diameter. Overlap the mushroom strips as you go. These are the base for the tarts.
3. Season each mushroom base with salt and pepper and sprinkle over a small amount of Emmental. The melted cheese will help to hold the mushroom base together. Grill for 3–4 minutes until the cheese is fully melted and the mushrooms have released some of their moisture.
4. Divide the spinach and pile it on to the tarts, then add the thyme leaves, a pinch of truffle salt and the remaining cheese.
5. Grill for a further 3–5 minutes until the cheese is bubbling, melted and deeply golden around the edges.
6. Leave the tarts to cool for 5 minutes to allow the cheese to firm up slightly.
7. Drizzle the rocket with the apple cider vinegar and a pinch of sea salt flakes and serve immediately.

CAULIFLOWER PIZZA

Cauliflower steaks are the perfect base for these little pizzas. The combination of pepper ketchup, oregano and melted cheese, bubbling and slightly scorched around the edges, is heavenly. Authentic pizzeria aromas will fill your kitchen and any pizza cravings will be fully alleviated! It's worth making a batch of pepper ketchup for this recipe alone. This recipe is not suitable for those avoiding nightshades.

SERVES 2
PREP: 5 MINUTES
COOK : 10 MINUTES

200g cauliflower slices, cut from 1 whole cauliflower (see steps 2 and 3)
4 tbsp Red Pepper Ketchup* (see page 56)
1 tsp dried oregano
160g Cheddar cheese, grated
sea salt and freshly ground black pepper

1. Preheat the oven to 230°C/210°C fan/gas mark 8.
2. Parboil the whole cauliflower for 8–10 minutes in salted water in a large saucepan. Drain and immediately immerse the cauliflower in cold water to stop the cooking process.
3. Use a large, sharp knife to cut the cauliflower into slices about 1–2cm thick.
4. Top the cauliflower slices with the ketchup, oregano and cheese.
5. Bake in the hot oven for 10 minutes until the cheese is slightly charred at the edges and melted in the middle.

TIP: *The cauliflower bases and pepper ketchup can be prepared in advance and frozen.*

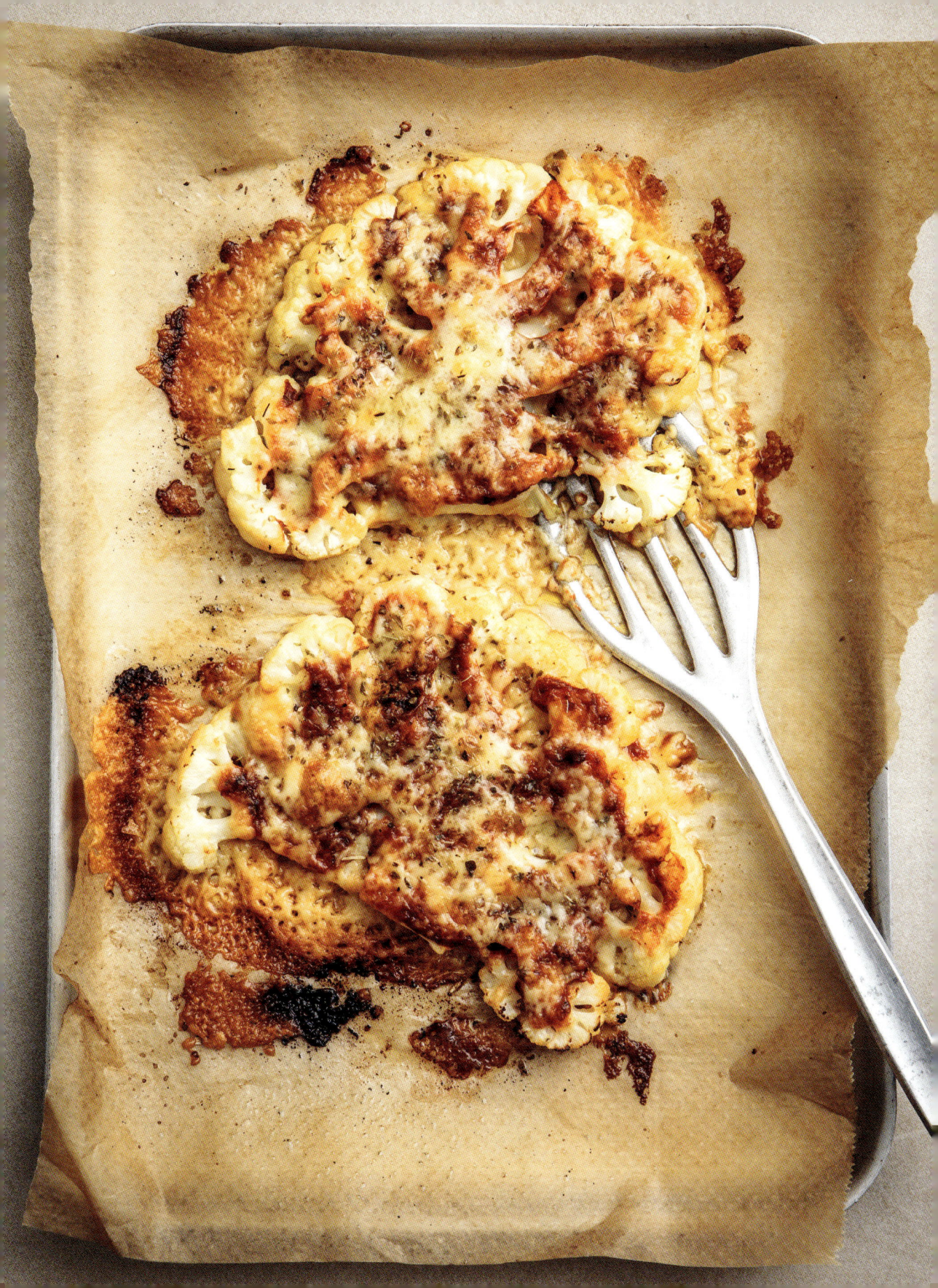

FRAGRANT STIR-FRIED STEAK

You need a good non-stick frying pan or wok for this recipe so you can heavily sear the beef. This process creates colour and umami depth. The addition of Chinese 5 spice, ginger and garlic brings the flavours of hoisin, making this a simple, quick dish full of punchy flavours.

SERVES 2
PREP: 10 MINUTES
COOK: 10 MINUTES

260g lean beef steak, cut into strips
50g onion, finely sliced
2 garlic cloves, finely sliced
1 tsp grated fresh ginger
¼ tsp Chinese 5 spice
¼ tsp chilli flakes* (optional)
1 tbsp tamari
60g broccoli, sliced into strips
50g carrot, julienned
50g green beans, halved
50g pak choi, chopped
fresh coriander, to serve

1. Heat a non-stick frying pan or wok over a medium–high heat, add the steak, and allow the meat to sear without stirring.
2. After 2–3 minutes, add the onion, garlic, ginger, Chinese 5 spice, chilli flakes (if using), tamari and a splash of water to deglaze the pan.
3. Add the broccoli, carrot and green beans. Stir and cover with a lid to allow the vegetables to briefly steam for 2–3 minutes.
4. Add the pak choi and cook uncovered for a further 1–2 minutes.
5. Serve with a scattering of fresh coriander.

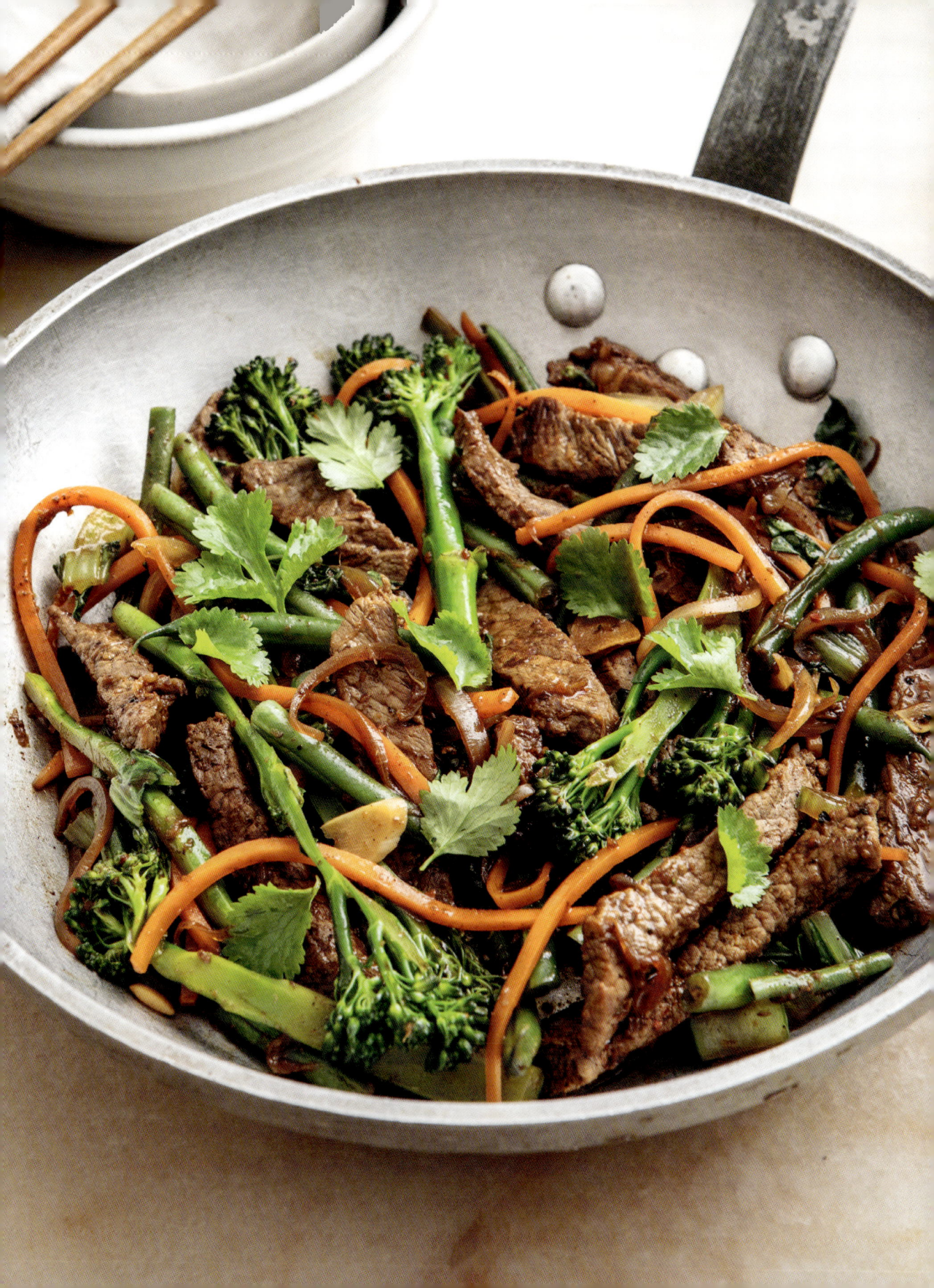

AMBROSIAL GARLIC BRAISED CHICKPEAS

Who knew that such humble ingredients could create such a deeply delicious bowl of comfort and joy? This really is a mellow, garlicky hug in a bowl – perfect for midweek suppers when you're tired, hungry and short of time and ingredients. Queen chickpeas in a jar are larger and softer than those from a tin; in this recipe, their gentle creaminess makes all the difference.

SERVES 2
PREP: 10 MINUTES
COOK: 20 MINUTES

100g shallot, finely chopped
100g carrot, finely diced
60g celery, finely chopped
300ml chicken or vegetable stock
4 large garlic cloves, thinly sliced
320g chickpeas, preferably large queen chickpeas from a jar (see above)
1–2 tbsp roughly chopped fresh flat-leaf parsley, to serve
sea salt and freshly ground black pepper

1. In a deep-sided frying pan or a wok, gently cook the shallot, carrot and celery in a splash of stock for 2–3 minutes to slightly soften.
2. Add the remainder of the stock, the garlic, chickpeas and a generous grind of salt and pepper. Simmer gently for about 20 minutes until the liquid has been absorbed or evaporated and all that's left in the pan are soft vegetables and chickpeas in a little syrupy sauce.
3. Serve with more freshly ground black pepper and a scattering of flat-leaf parsley.

TIP: *Freezes well and is great for batch cooking.*

LENTIL RAGU WITH RICE

This is a deliciously warming and savoury vegan recipe. I serve it with vegetable rice, but it is also yummy served with spiralised vegetables. It's a good recipe to batch cook and freeze, so you are prepared for days when you're short on time and have a hungry family to feed. For a friends and family version, serve with wholewheat pasta or brown rice.

SERVES 2
PREP: 10 MINUTES
COOK: 25 MINUTES

40g onion, finely diced
30g carrot, finely diced
30g mushrooms, finely sliced
350ml fresh vegetable stock
10g/2 tsp tomato purée* (optional)
2 garlic cloves, crushed
2–3 sprigs of fresh thyme
1 bay leaf
260g cooked brown or green lentils
150g cauliflower rice (see page 140)
sea salt and freshly ground white pepper

1. In a saucepan cook the onion, carrot and mushrooms in a splash of stock for 5 minutes to soften, then add the tomato purée (if using) and cook for a further minute.
2. Add the garlic, remaining stock, the thyme and bay leaf and some salt and pepper. Simmer over a low heat for about 10–15 minutes until the stock has reduced and thickened slightly and the vegetables are completely soft.
3. Add the lentils and continue to simmer for a few minutes to warm them through.
4. Remove the bay leaf and thyme, taste and season with salt and pepper.
5. Cook the cauliflower rice in a splash of water for about 2–3 minutes, drain and serve immediately with the ragu.

> **VARIATION**
> - Replace the tomato purée with 10g of extra mushrooms if you are avoiding nightshades.

STIR-FRIED TOFU, PAK CHOI & BROCCOLI WITH GINGER & GARLIC

As a relatively bland source of excellent plant protein, tofu lends itself brilliantly to a marinade. It absorbs all and any flavours you throw at it! Here, the classic Chinese flavours of soy, garlic, ginger and 5 spice work together to create a deliciously fragrant stir fry. The tofu is sliced into batons to give a larger surface area, so it soaks up and takes on all the wonderful, aromatic flavours.

SERVES 2
PREP: 10 MINUTES (PLUS 30 MINUTES–2 HOURS MARINADING)
COOK: 10 MINUTES

2 tbsp tamari
3 garlic cloves, crushed
2 tsp finely grated fresh ginger
1½ tsp Chinese 5 spice
260g firm organic tofu, sliced into slim batons
60g onion, finely chopped
100g pak choi, roughly chopped
80g tenderstem broccoli, sliced lengthways
20g spring onion, finely sliced lengthways
chopped fresh coriander, to serve

1. To prepare the marinade, mix the tamari, garlic, ginger and 5 spice in a bowl. Add the tofu and mix until it is thoroughly coated. Refrigerate and leave to marinate for a minimum of 30 minutes and a maximum of 2 hours.
2. Put a wok or frying pan over a medium heat and cook the tofu and onion for 5–6 minutes in a splash of water.
3. Turn up the heat and add the pak choi and broccoli. Cook for a further 5 minutes, stirring regularly, until the vegetables are slightly wilted and softened. Be careful not to break up the tofu pieces as you stir.
4. Serve immediately with the spring onion and chopped coriander.

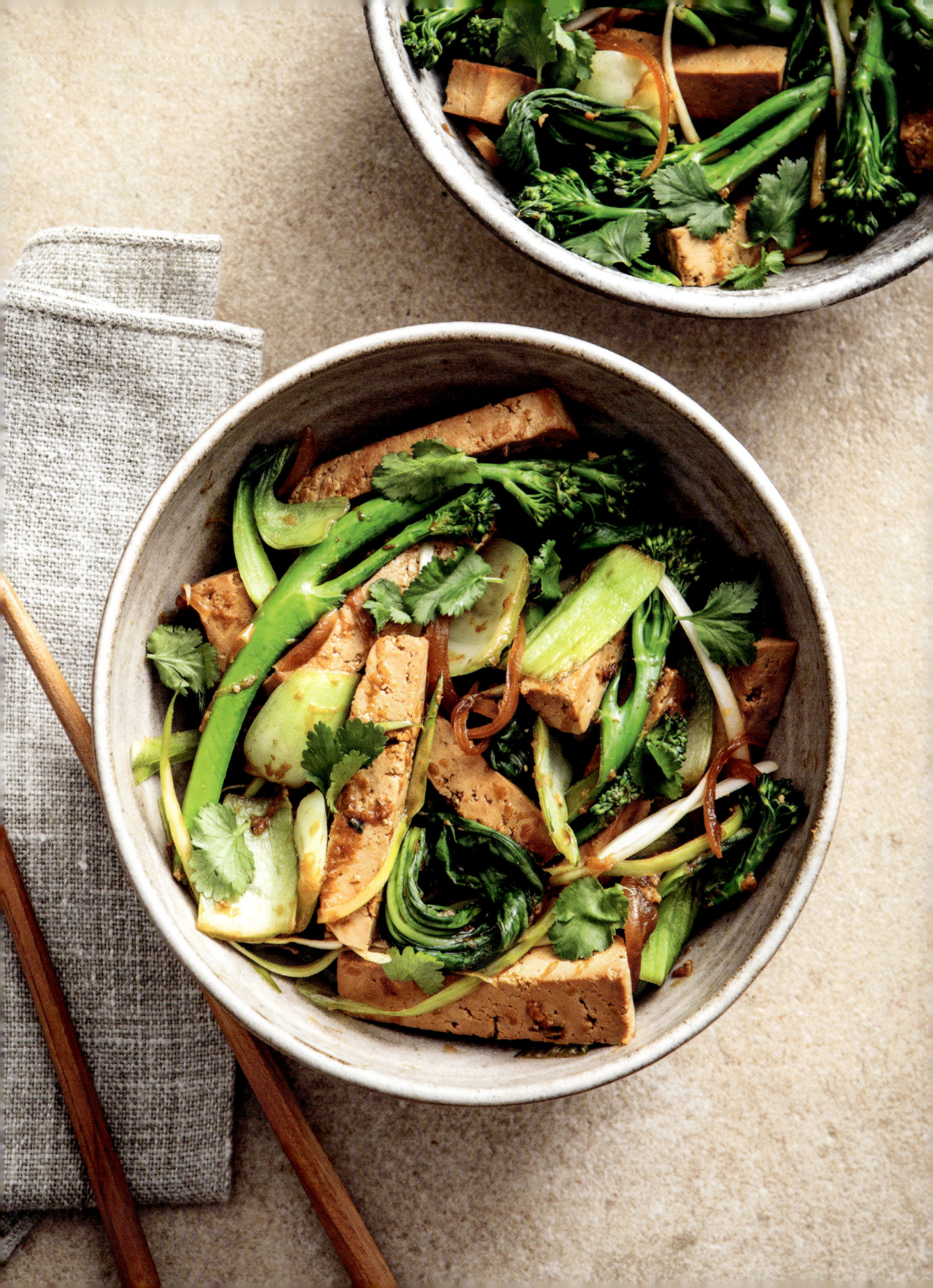

Good To Go

CRAB SLIDERS

You have full permission to spoil yourself during Reset and delicate white crab meat certainly is an indulgence. I often treat myself to these little beauties during my second Reset weekend – they're a little prize for doing so well, perfect on a Saturday night with a glass of HBD champagne. Most joyous of all is that there is no cooking involved and barely any washing up. The sliders are inspired by the divine crab toasts from my favourite London riverside restaurant. Bitter chicory leaves balance the sweet flavours of the crab, while peppery radish and cool cucumber add crunch.

SERVES 2
PREP: 10 MINUTES

- 260g white crab meat
- 20g spring onion, finely chopped
- 60g cucumber, peeled, deseeded and very finely diced
- 30g radishes, very finely diced
- 1 tbsp finely chopped fresh chives
- zest and juice of 1 lemon,
- ¼ tsp chilli flakes* (optional)
- 150g red or white chicory leaves, whole
- sea salt and freshly ground black pepper

1. In a medium-sized bowl, mix the crab, spring onion, cucumber, radish and chives.
2. Season the mixture with the lemon zest and juice, chilli flakes (if using) and salt and pepper. Mix well.
3. Pile the crab mixture into the chicory leaves to serve.

> **VARIATION**
> - If you are avoiding nightshades, replace the chilli flakes with a generous pinch of white pepper.

PRAWN & MANGO SUMMER ROLLS

These pretty summer rolls are a flavour sensation made with simple, fresh ingredients and a perfect example of the whole being *so* much greater than the sum of its parts! Every flavour and texture enhances and elevates the next; the result is summery magic. The combination of tropical mango, sweet meaty prawns and creamy avocado is classic. The addition of citrussy coriander, crisp lettuce and cool cucumber balances the sweet elements perfectly.

SERVES 2
PREP: 15 MINUTES

160g cucumber ribbons (see step 1)
260g king prawns, roughly chopped
2 tbsp roughly chopped fresh coriander
1 green chilli* (optional)
70g avocado, thinly sliced
30g lettuce (iceberg or similar), shredded
140g fresh mango, thinly sliced
sea salt and freshly ground black pepper

1. To make wafer-thin cucumber ribbons suitable for rolling, repeatedly run a potato peeler down the length of a cucumber.
2. On a sheet of parchment paper or foil, overlap the ribbons to create an oblong sheet to use as a wrapper.
3. Combine the prawns, coriander, a grind of salt and pepper and the green chilli (if using) in a bowl.
4. Lay the avocado slices across the length of the cucumber wrapper about a third of the way up. Top the avocado with the shredded lettuce and then the mango. Finish by spooning the prawn mixture on top of the mango layer.
5. Use the parchment paper or foil to roll up as tightly as possible, much as you would a sausage roll.
6. Slice and serve immediately. Or you can wrap the rolls tightly in foil or an airtight container and keep them chilled to eat later that day.

TIP: *This recipe only calls for 140g of mango, but feel free to eat the remaining 60g from your allowance for dessert!*

VARIATION
- If you know you are OK with nightshades, green chilli* is a great addition to these rolls. I always have fresh chillies in the freezer to finely grate from frozen as desired.

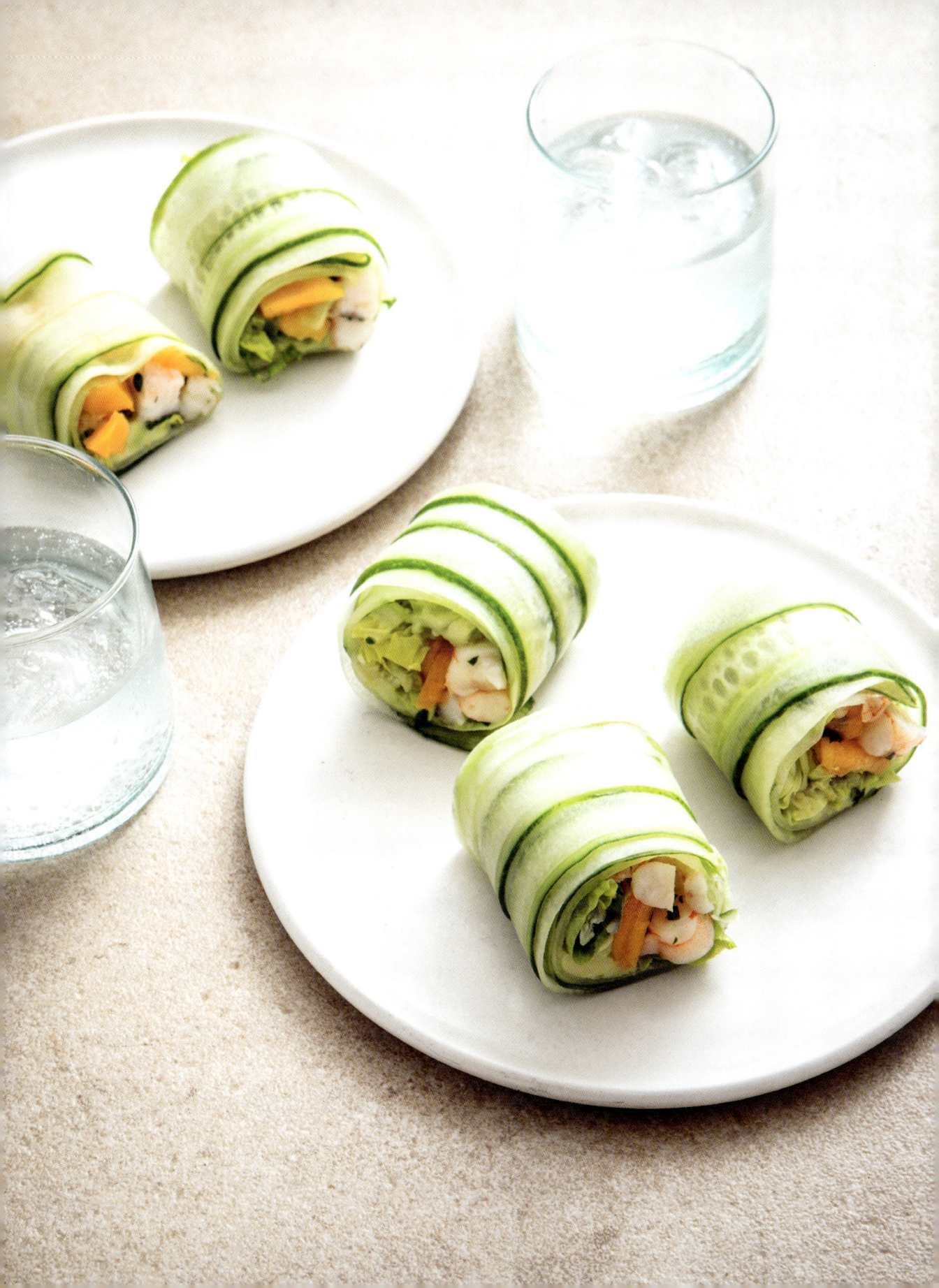

TUNA SUSHI

These gorgeous little sushi rolls are so easy to make and perfect for a speedy packed lunch. Seaweed is a powerhouse of nutrients and minerals which, when combined with fresh raw vegetables and oily fish, creates a delicious and supremely nutritious meal.

SERVES 2
PREP: 15 MINUTES

260g tinned tuna, in spring water or brine
2 tsp tamari
1 tsp minced fresh ginger
3–4 tbsp finely chopped fresh coriander
30g spring onion, finely chopped
10g/4–5 nori seaweed wrappers
80g cucumber, julienned
90g carrot, finely julienned
50g red cabbage, shredded

1. Combine the tuna, tamari, ginger, coriander and spring onion in a bowl and mix well.
2. Lay a sheet of nori on a sushi rolling mat. If you don't have one a piece of foil or parchment works well.
3. Put about a quarter of the tuna mixture in a sausage shape across the width of the nori wrapper, about a third of the way up. Spread a layer of cucumber, carrot and red cabbage on top of the tuna.
4. Roll up the wrapper as firmly as possible, in the way you would roll a sausage roll. Repeat with the remaining wrappers and tuna mixture.
5. Slice the rolls into sections. Refrigerate and eat within 24 hours.

VARIATION
- These rolls are a brilliant vessel for any combination of fish and seafood. They are delicious made with tofu, crab or salmon.

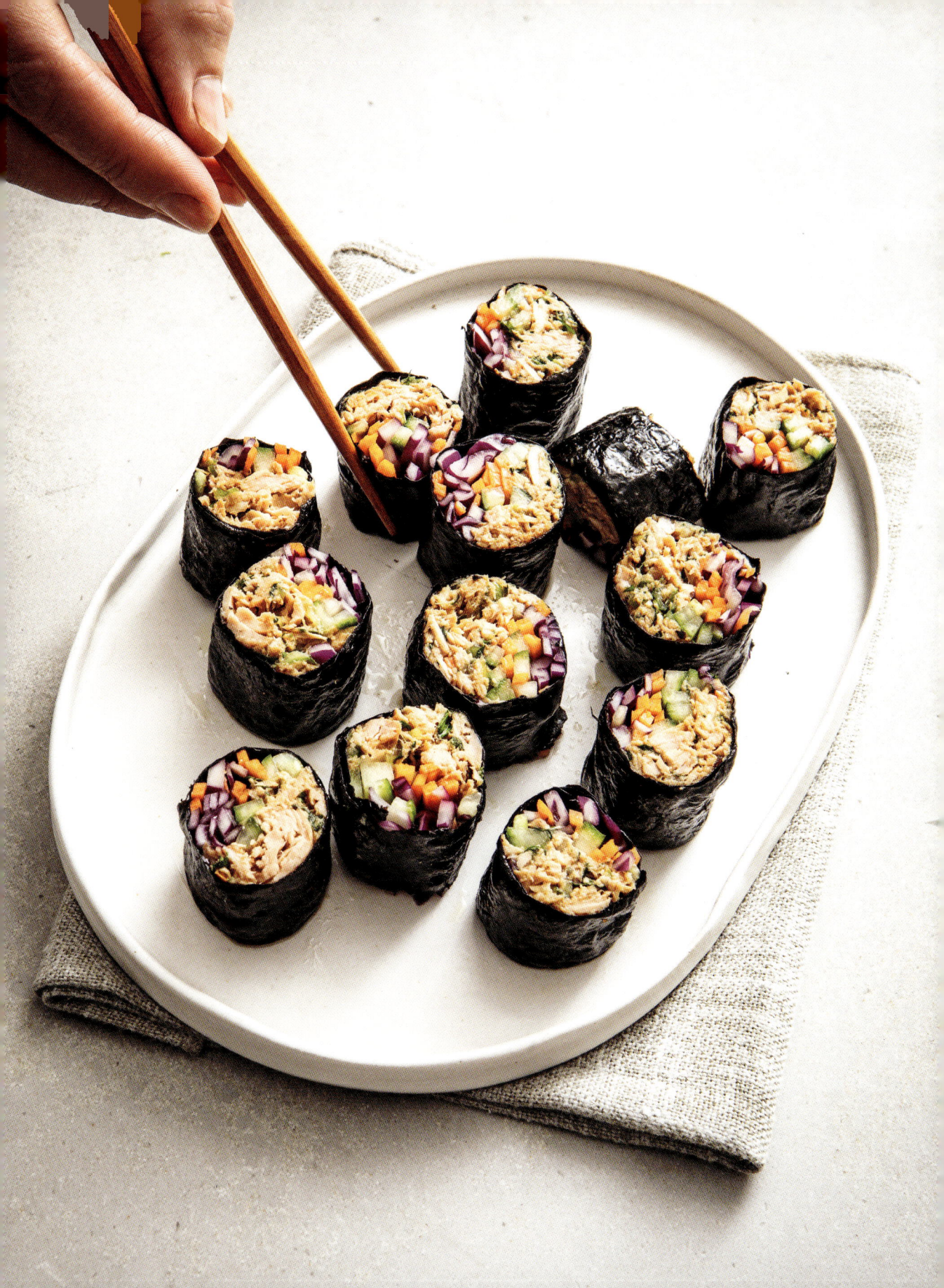

CHICKEN SATAY SLIDERS WITH CREAMY AVOCADO

These sizzling chicken skewers are fragrant with lemongrass, ginger and garlic. They balance wonderfully with the cool, creamy avocado and crisp little gem.

SERVES 2
PREP: 15 MINUTES
COOK: 15 MINUTES

FOR THE CHICKEN SATAY
3 garlic cloves, chopped
1 stalk of lemongrass, chopped
2 tsp chopped fresh ginger
1 small, mild green chilli*, chopped
2 tbsp chopped fresh coriander stalks and leaves
20g spring onion, chopped
260g chicken mince
sea salt

FOR THE AVOCADO CREAM
120g ripe avocado
1 tbsp lemon juice
1 small, mild green chilli*, finely chopped
2 garlic cloves, crushed
80g (8) whole little gem lettuce leaves, to serve
40g spring onion, sliced, to serve
sea salt and freshly ground black pepper

1. Preheat the oven to 180°C/160°C fan/gas mark 4.
2. Soak 8 small (15cm) bamboo skewers in water for a minimum of 10 minutes; this prevents them from burning. (Alternatively, use metal skewers.)
3. Make the satay paste. Put the garlic, lemongrass, ginger, green chilli (if using), coriander, spring onion and a generous pinch of sea salt in a blender and pulse to form a smooth paste. Alternatively, this can be done by hand in a pestle and mortar. Add the spice paste to the chicken mince and mix thoroughly.
4. Divide the spiced mince into 8 equal-sized sausage shapes. Press a skewer into each sausage, pushing the mince tightly around each one to create a long kofta style kebab.
5. Put the skewers on a non-stick baking sheet and cook in the preheated oven for 6–7 minutes. Flip them over and continue to cook for a further 6–7 minutes until the juices run clear.
6. Meanwhile, thoroughly mash the avocado, add the lemon juice, green chilli (if using) and crushed garlic. Season with salt and pepper and mix well until creamy, adding a splash of cold water to loosen the mixture if necessary.
7. To assemble, divide the creamy avocado mixture between the lettuce leaves. Top each one with a chicken skewer and garnish with spring onion and coriander.

VARIATION
- If you are avoiding nightshades, replace the green chilli with a generous pinch of white pepper.

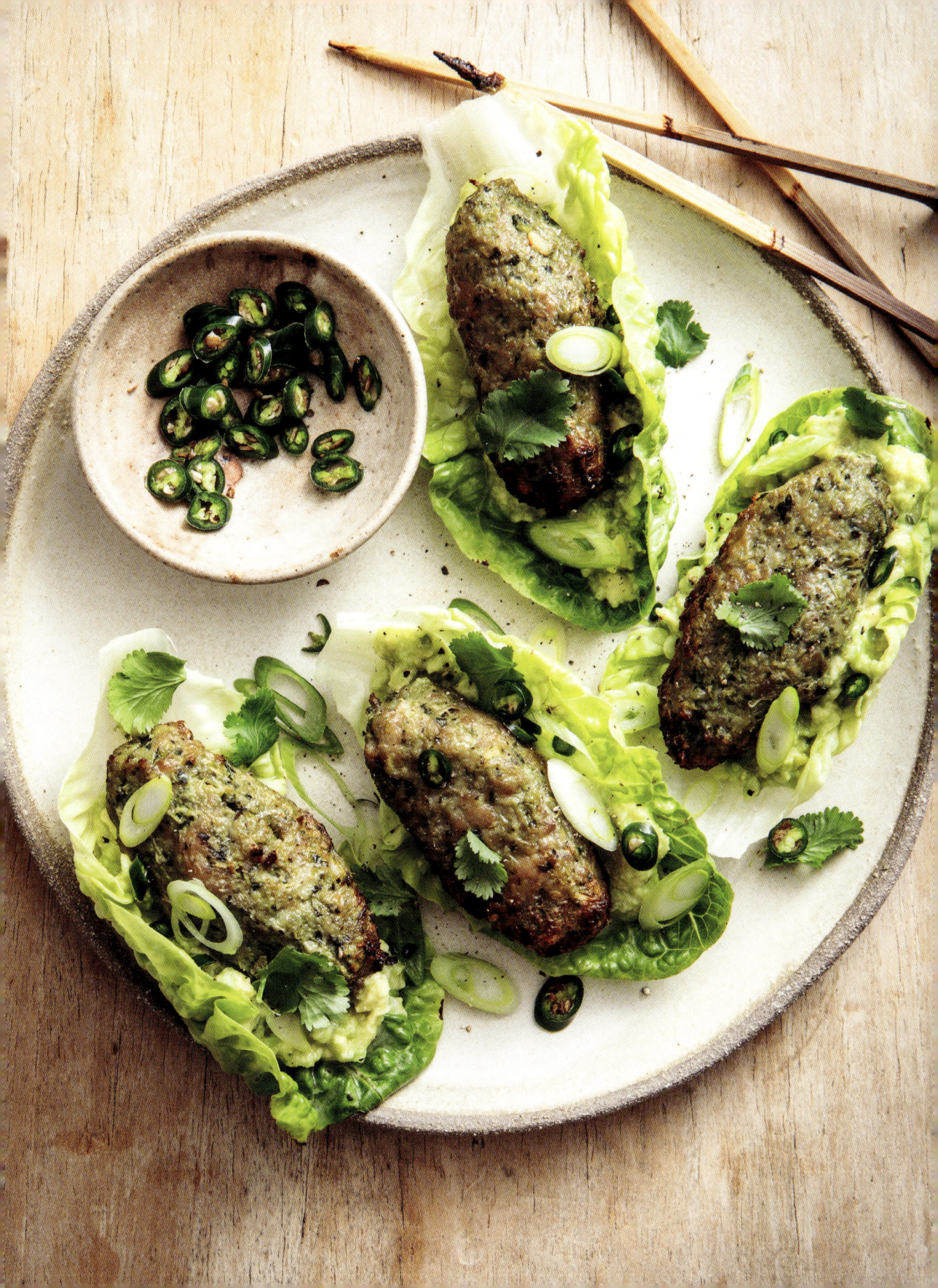

SMOKED MACKEREL PATE WITH QUICK PICKLES

Rich, oily smoked mackerel is jam packed with omegas and delicious when flaked and seasoned and made into a pate. The quick pickled vegetables, sweetly sharp and zesty, cut through the richness of the fish beautifully.

SERVES 2
PREP: 15 MINUTES (PLUS 15–60 MINUTES STEEPING)

FOR THE QUICK PICKLED VEGETABLES
40g cucumber, cut into thin batons
40g radishes, sliced
2 tsp finely chopped fresh dill
1–2 tbsp apple cider vinegar
sea salt

FOR THE PATE
260g smoked mackerel, skin removed and flesh flaked
30g red onion, finely sliced
zest and juice of 1 lemon
2–3 tbsp chopped fresh coriander
freshly ground black pepper
150g crudites of choice, to serve

1. First make the pickled vegetables. Combine the cucumber, radish, dill, apple cider vinegar and a pinch of salt in a bowl. Leave to steep for 15 minutes to 1 hour.
2. Meanwhile, combine the mackerel, red onion, lemon zest and juice, coriander and black pepper in a bowl and mix well.
3. Drain the pickled vegetables and serve with the pate and crudites of your choice.

LEMON & CORIANDER HUMMUS WITH CRUDITES

I was happily surprised to discover that hummus without both the tahini and olive oil can still be rather delicious! To maximise flavour, I've added lemon and coriander, but feel free to omit both for a more traditional hummus, or experiment with your own flavour combinations. Add herbs, roasted veggies and spices of your own; it's time to get creative!

SERVES 2
PREP: 10 MINUTES

320g cooked chickpeas
2 garlic cloves, crushed
2 tsp lemon juice
3–4 tbsp cold water
2 tbsp very finely chopped fresh coriander
1 tbsp lemon zest
260g veggie crudites of your choice
sea salt and freshly ground black pepper

1. Put the chickpeas, garlic, lemon juice, a pinch of salt and pepper and the cold water in a food processor and purée until smooth and silky. Add more water if necessary until you have the perfect dipping consistency.
2. Stir in the coriander and lemon zest, taste and season with more salt and pepper if necessary.
3. Serve with a selection of crudites.

TRICOLORE WRAP

Tricolore salad represents the colours of the Italian flag and bursts with classic Italian flavours. Eating creamy, cool mozzarella feels a treat and the sweet peppers more than make up for the limited quantity of tomato and – of course – there must be basil. These wraps are perfect to eat out and about; the crunchy outer iceberg lettuce leaves work brilliantly as a wrapper for the filling.

SERVES 2
PREP: 10 MINUTES

120g whole outer leaves of iceberg lettuce
40g rocket
40g fresh tomato*, sliced
60g roasted red pepper*, thinly sliced into strips
160g mozzarella, sliced
2–3 tbsp fresh basil leaves, torn
sea salt and freshly ground black pepper

1. Make two piles of lettuce, spreading the leaves out into a rough oblong shape; these will be your wrappers.
2. Lay the rocket, tomato and pepper slices down the middle of each wrap, top with the mozzarella, a grind of salt and pepper and the torn basil.
3. Roll up each wrap as tightly as possible, much as you would a sausage roll.
4. Eat immediately or wrap in a strip of parchment and secure with a cocktail stick.

VARIATION
- Be creative with the fillings: if you're avoiding nightshades, cold chicken or hummus and avocado work well.

TIP: *To hold the wrap together, fix a strip of baking parchment around it and secure with a wooden toothpick. This is useful when making a packed lunch or picnic.*

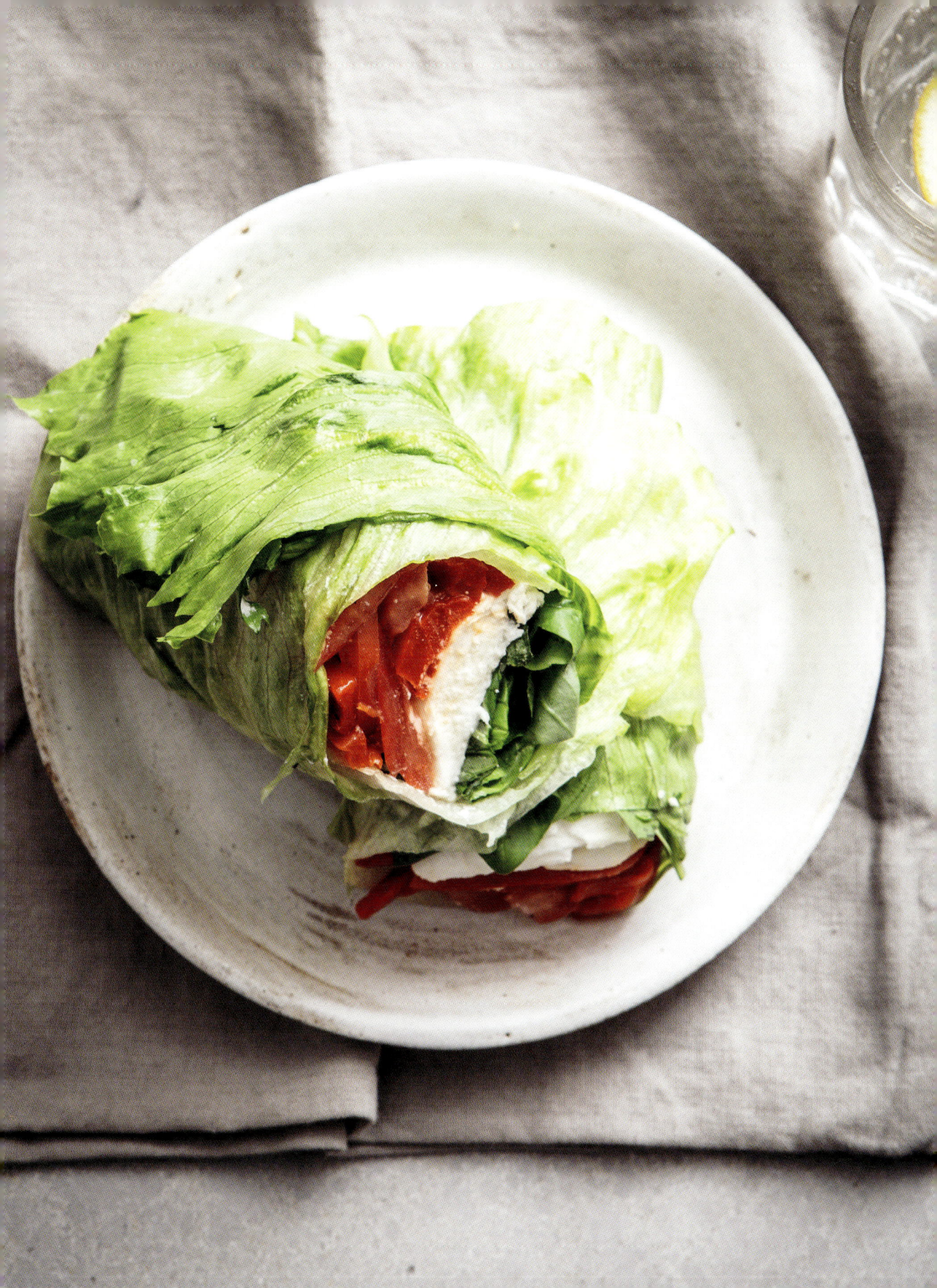

FETA WITH LEVANTINE TABBOULEH

It never ceases to amaze me how deliciously moreish this tabbouleh salad is. The blitzed broccoli gives extra freshness and bite, while the lemon, parsley and punchy red onion make it fresh and zingy with a citrus kick. Creamy, rich feta is the perfect accompaniment to the vibrant tabbouleh; alternatively, try it with chicken or fish.

SERVES 2
PREP: 15 MINUTES

130g broccoli stems
50g cherry tomatoes*, finely chopped
50g red pepper*, finely chopped
30g red onion, finely chopped
zest and juice of 1 lemon,
3 tbsp chopped fresh flat-leaf parsley
160g feta, crumbled
sea salt and freshly ground black pepper

1. Roughly chop the broccoli stems and briefly blitz them in a food processor to create broccoli rice.
2. Put the tomatoes, red pepper, red onion, lemon zest and juice and the parsley into a bowl. Add the broccoli and a generous pinch of salt and pepper and stir well.
3. Serve with the feta crumbled on top.

VARIATION
- If you are avoiding nightshades, swap the red pepper and tomatoes for finely chopped celery and cucumber.

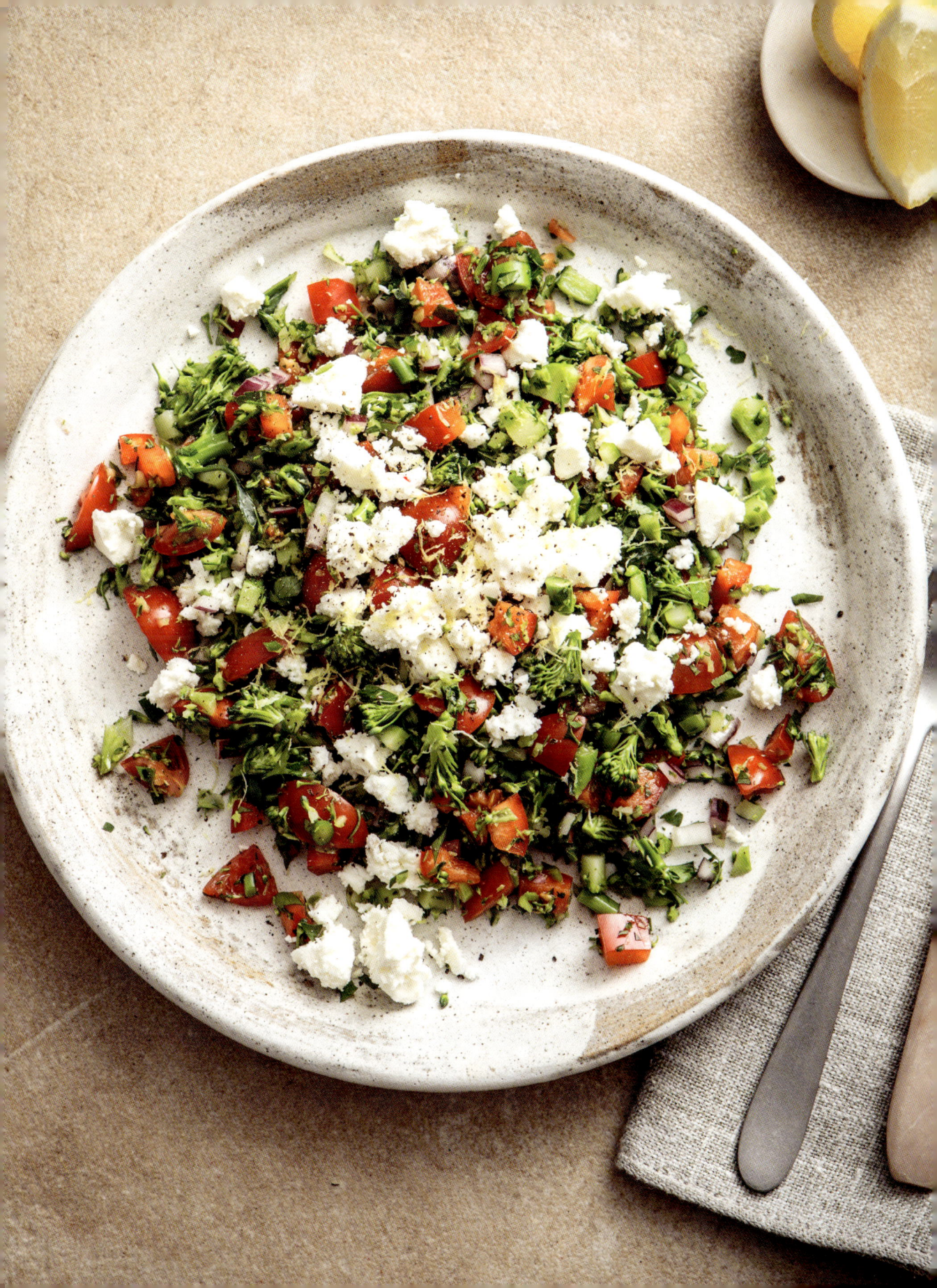

DAY 17 THE RESULTS OF YOUR RESET – HUGE CHANGES AND A *HUGE* ACHIEVEMENT!

You've proved to yourself that:

- You can go for five hours or longer without eating (and without keeling over!)
- You don't need snacks or sugar to give you energy – your energy's never been better
- You've stabilised your blood sugar and got insulin back under control
- Your body *can* burn fat for energy
- You've got used to drinking water
- You've got used to smaller portions
- You've killed the wine/sugar monster
- You've got used to drinking black tea/coffee
- You're no longer hungry
- You've turned from a sugar burner into a fat burner!
- You've got your joy and your mojo back
- You can't wait to get going with Phase 3
- You've laid the new foundations and you're building a new body. You've just begun, but you've completed the toughest part. You've broken the habits of a lifetime – you're in charge now and it feels great. *Congratulations!*

A BRIEF LOOK AHEAD TO PHASE 3

This is where HBD feasting comes in with weekly treat meals! Extra virgin olive oil is added too for its incredible health-giving properties. You'll have an expanded food list with optional rye bread and starchier vegetables, including celeriac, beetroot, parsnips and sweet potatoes. Miso, a superfood, can be enjoyed with soy based meals in Phase 3. And, joy of joys, dark chocolate!

Treat yourself to *The HBD Cookbook* for lots of Phase 3 and Phase 4 recipes, but meanwhile you'll have enough for the first week or few days in Phase 3 here if you add a tablespoon of extra virgin olive oil to Phase 2 recipes.

Community: The HBD Club

I've often been asked if I plan to train HBD coaches, who would be professionally endorsed and enabled to coach others in HBD, and the answer is always no. And this is why.

My overarching motivation and my mission for putting what I have learned in years of clinical experience into The Human Being Diet, is to empower you with the knowledge you need to become your own best nutritionist. So you can become your own best and most trusted guide and coach. My aim is to demystify nutrition and to ensure that you find the very best diet or way of eating for *you* as a biochemically unique individual. I also aim to help you understand how to decode the messages from your body and to nurture yourself in the way that suits you best.

You don't need anyone to help you do this – in fact nobody but you can do this work – the power is in your hands alone. HBD is a voyage of self-discovery, and only *you* can discover how you react, in body and mind, to any particular foods or combinations of foods. That's my mission – to enable and empower you to best look after your own health.

HBD is about going within and learning to trust and nurture yourself with love and self-respect. It can be difficult to embrace self-love, but it grows easier with time, and with age and with practice. An important part of this process of self-nurture is in preparing and cooking food for yourself – and Lizzie shows you how! You do not need to be a talented cook to get great results and to enjoy delicious and nourishing food – just follow the recipes here.

All the information you need for success is in my first book, *The Human Being Diet*. The cookbooks, *The HBD Cookbook* and this one of course, ensure that you can have the most deliciously nutritious experience while you are feasting and fasting your way to great energy and health. A lovely woman on Instagram aptly described The Human Being Diet as 'the rules' and the cookbooks as 'the tools'.

We all understand the power of community and while one-to-one coaching is the antithesis of the fundamental HBD values, community is all important. In the early days the HBD gang on Instagram was a friendly, tight-knit community but it expanded quickly and eventually its warm and generous vibe – the feeling of us all being in it together – was diluted. Some set up Facebook groups that are leading to confusion for HBD followers. I am asked if they are 'offical'. My reply is that 'if it hasn't got my name on it it's not HBD'.

That's why we created The HBD Club. We needed an official place for motivation, inspiration and support, where people could learn more about the programme and find official answers to their questions. It's a community of generous people who want the best for each other and themselves and where no one feels alone. We hope to see you there!

ACKNOWLEDGEMENTS

PETRONELLA
With thanks to Katya Shipster and her team at HarperCollins for creating this beautiful cookbook to add to our flourishing HBD collection. To Lizzie for her dazzlingly delicious recipes and enthusiasm for this book. And as ever and always thanks to my darling husband Riccardo for his invaluable advice and support.

LIZZIE
Huge thanks to my family and friends for your love, patience and encouragement. To my taste testers and cheerleaders, the Whiting/Compston/Le Bon families for being there every step of the way; with special thanks thanks to Kit for her invaluable help and to Yasmin for being our shoot stylist extraordinaire. Finally, the biggest thanks must go to Petronella for trusting me with her magical HBD larder and for all her warmth, generosity and wisdom.

NOTES

1. Iacobucci, G. 'GLP-1 agonists: 82 deaths linked to adverse reactions, UK data show.' *BMJ* 2025; 388 :r390 doi:10.1136/bmj.r390

2. Gorgojo-Martínez, JJ, et al. 'Clinical Recommendations to Manage Gastrointestinal Adverse Events in Patients Treated with Glp-1 Receptor Agonists: A Multidisciplinary Expert Consensus.' *J Clin Med*. 2022 Dec 24;12(1):145. doi: 10.3390/jcm12010145. PMID: 36614945; PMCID: PMC9821052.

3. The Cleveland Clinic, 'GLP-1 Agonists'. (https://my.clevelandclinic.org/health/treatments/13901-glp-1-agonists)

4. Rodriguez, PJ, et al. Discontinuation and Reinitiation of Dual-Labeled GLP-1 Receptor Agonists Among US Adults With Overweight or Obesity. *JAMA Netw Open*. 2025;8(1):e2457349. doi:10.1001/jamanetworkopen.2024.57349

INDEX

A
acetic acid 43
acid reflux 24
additives 20
adipocytes 37
air fryers 53
allergies: dairy foods 32
   oral allergy syndrome 45
Ambrosial Garlic Braised Chickpeas 192
amino acids 30–1
ammonia 31
antibiotics 17
antibodies, autoimmune 24
antioxidants 29, 45, 46
apple cider vinegar 10, 36, 43, 69, 99, 106
   Chimichurri Dressing 57
   Creamy Avocado Dressing 88
   Mango Chutney 61
   Mustard Dressing 59
   Quick Pickles 204
apples 45
   Apple & Pumpkin Spiced Crumble Pots 122
   Breakfast Slaw 110
   Carrot & Ginger Muffins 128
   Scandi Mackerel Salad 162
   Sweet & Sour Salmon 156
Aromatic Baked Bass en Papillote 184
artichokes 45
asparagus 45
   Asparagus, Courgette & Herb Frittata 126
   Smash Burgers with Fondant Onion 138
aubergines 33
   Baba Ganoush 149
   Caponata with Cod 153
   Moussaka 145
autoimmune disorders 11, 24
avocados 46
   Avocado & Smoked Salmon Salad 113
   Avocado Cream 202
   Creamy Avocado Dressing 88
   Mango Salsa 154
   Prawn & Mango Summer Rolls 198
   Shredded Chicken & Tarragon Salad 120
   Spicy Guacamole 136
   Tomato Carpaccio with Avocado, Red Onion & Basil 84

B
Baba Ganoush 149
bacteria, gut microbiome 20, 25, 29, 49
Bake-O-Glide 53
Baked Green Eggs 129
Baked Sea Bream with Mash & Greens 181
basil: Pistou 58
   Tomato Carpaccio with Avocado, Red Onion & Basil 84
   Tricolore Wrap 206
batch cooking 35
baths, Epsom salt 74
beans (dried) 30, 31
   see also butter beans
beef: Bolognese 161
   Chilli Beef Tacos 160
   Classic Beef Stew with Thyme 166
   Fragrant Stir-fried Steak 190
   Smash Burgers with Fondant Onion 138
the Best Chicken Bone Stock 62
bile 70
binge eating 24
bloating 32, 43
blood pressure 24, 48
blood sugar levels 10, 20, 30, 40, 43
body measurements 75
Bolognese 161

brain 38
bread 23, 30, 106
  Flatbreads 178
breakfast 30, 102, 109–29
Breakfast Slaw 110
broccoli 45
  Baked Green Eggs 129
  Feta with Levantine Tabbouleh 208
  Fragrant Stir-fried Steak 190
  Pomegranate Couscous 146
  Stir-fried Tofu, Pak Choi & Broccoli with Ginger & Garlic 194
Broth, Steaming Hungarian Meatball 170
brown fat 45
buckwheat 30
burgers: Smash Burgers with Fondant Onion 138
butter beans: Butter Bean Cream 176
  Smokie Veggie Goulash 176
butternut squash: Apple & Pumpkin Spiced Crumble Pots 122
  Bolognese 161
  Butternut Squash & Green Bean Curry 87
  Butternut Squash & Sage Risotto 171
  Butternut Squash, Turmeric & Ginger Soup 80
  Chana Masala with Flatbreads 178
  Chicken & Pomegranate Tagine with Saffron Couscous 152
  Curry Sauce 60
  Jambalaya 139
  Moroccan Lamb Casserole with Squash & Spinach 172
  Smokie Veggie Goulash 176
  Smoky Tofu Hash 124
  Sunshine Saffron Cauliflower Rice Pilau 86

C

cabbage 45
  Baked Green Eggs 129
  Breakfast Slaw 110
  Cabbage Leaf Gyozas 133
  Classic Beef Stew with Thyme 166
  Garlic Braised Hispi Cabbage with Caramelised Onions 90
  Steaming Hungarian Meatball Broth 170
  see also red cabbage
calcium 29
calories 20, 34–5
Caponata with Cod 153
carbohydrates 29–30
cardamom pods: Mango Chutney 61
cardio exercise 22
carrots: Ambrosial Garlic Braised Chickpeas 192
  Aromatic Baked Bass en Papillote 184
  the Best Chicken Bone Stock 62
  Breakfast Slaw 110
  Carrot & Ginger Muffins 128
  Chilli Beef Tacos 160
  Classic Beef Stew with Thyme 166
  Classic Vegetable Stock 63
  Fragrant Stir-fried Steak 190
  Lentil Ragu with Rice 193
  Rainbow Slaw with Creamy Avocado Dressing 88
  Steaming Hungarian Meatball Broth 170
  Sunshine Saffron Cauliflower Rice Pilau 86
  Thai-style Ramen 78
  Tuna Sushi 200
casein 32
casseroles *see* stews and casseroles
cauliflower 45
  Baked Sea Bream with Mash & Greens 181
  Cauliflower & Roasted Garlic Soup 82
  Cauliflower Pizza 188
cauliflower rice: Chicken Cauliflower Rice Pilaf 186
  Kedgeree 134
  King Prawn Paella 140
  Lentil Ragu with Rice 193
  Saffron Couscous 152
  Sunshine Saffron Cauliflower Rice Pilau 86
  Tempeh Chilli with Cauliflower Rice 177
celery 45
  Smoked Mackerel Sushi 116
  Steaming Hungarian Meatball Broth 170
  Waldorf Salad 112

Chana Masala with Flatbreads 178
chard: Smoked Haddock & Wilted Greens 121
  Smoky Tofu Hash 124
cheese 32, 97
  Baked Feta Parcels 150
  Cauliflower Pizza 188
  Feta with Levantine Tabbouleh 208
  Greek Salad 117
  Halloumi, Strawberry & Mint Salad 118
  Parmesan Crisps 174
  Tricolore Wrap 206
  Truffle Mushroom Tarts with Emmental 187
chicken: the Best Chicken Bone Stock 62
  Braised Chicken with Fondant Leeks & Fennel 165
  Chicken & Pomegranate Tagine with Saffron Couscous 152
  Chicken Cauliflower Rice Pilaf 186
  Chicken Satay Sliders with Creamy Avocado 202
  Chicken Shawarma with Greek Salad 158
  Shredded Chicken & Tarragon Salad 120
  Spring Chicken Casserole 144
chickpea (gram) flour: Flatbreads 178
  Socca Bread 106
chickpea rice 105
  Butternut Squash & Sage Risotto 171
  Shiitake Mushroom, Spinach & Thyme Risotto 142
chickpeas 30, 31
  Ambrosial Garlic Braised Chickpeas 192
  Chana Masala with Flatbreads 178
  Lemon & Coriander Hummus with Crudites 205
chicory: Crab Sliders 197
  Scandi Mackerel Salad 162
chilli flakes: Tempeh Chilli with Cauliflower Rice 177
chillies: Avocado Cream 202
  Chicken Satay Sliders with Creamy Avocado 202
  Chilli Beef Tacos 160
  Mango Salsa 154
  Prawn & Mango Summer Rolls 198
  Sweet & Sour Salmon 156
Chimichurri Dressing 57
chives: Chimichurri Dressing 57
chloride 72

chlorogenic acid 45
chocolate 23
cholesterol 24, 43, 46
chromium 30
Chutney, Mango 61
cider vinegar see apple cider vinegar
circadian rhythm 38
Circle 17
Classic Beef Stew with Thyme 166
Classic Vegetable Stock 63
cod 46
  Caponata with Cod 153
coffee 22, 42, 65, 95, 99, 104
condiments 52
  Chimichurri Dressing 57
  Mango Chutney 61
  Mustard Dressing 59
  Pistou 58
  Red Pepper Ketchup 56
coriander: Chimichurri Dressing 57
  Lemon & Coriander Hummus with Crudites 205
cortisol 22, 49, 96
courgettes 45
  Aromatic Baked Bass en Papillote 184
  Asparagus, Courgette & Herb Frittata 126
  Baked Feta Parcels 150
  Caponata with Cod 153
  Carrot & Ginger Muffins 128
  Italian Pork & Fennel Meatballs 168
  Lemon & Rosemary Monkfish Skewers 182
  Moussaka 145
  Pistou Soup with Parmesan Crisps 174
  Spring Chicken Casserole 144
couscous: Pomegranate Couscous 146
  Saffron Couscous 152
cows' milk 32
Crab Sliders 197
cravings 10, 38, 43
Creamy Avocado Dressing 88
Crispy Fish Tacos with Spicy Guacamole 136
Crispy Sea Bass with Mango Salsa 154
Crudites, Lemon & Coriander Hummus with 205

cucumber: Avocado & Smoked Salmon Salad 113
  Crab Sliders 197
  Cucumber, Grape & Dill Salad with Tzatziki 114
  Greek Salad 117, 158
  Halloumi, Strawberry & Mint Salad 118
  Pomegranate Couscous 146
  Prawn & Mango Summer Rolls 198
  Quick Pickles 204
  Scandi Mackerel Salad 162
  Shredded Chicken & Tarragon Salad 120
  Smoked Mackerel Sushi 116
  Tomato Carpaccio with Avocado, Red Onion & Basil 84
  Tuna Sushi 200
  Tzatziki 114
  Waldorf Salad 112
curry: Butternut Squash & Green Bean Curry 87
  Chana Masala with Flatbreads 178
  Curry Sauce 60
  Kedgeree 134

D

dairy foods 27, 30, 31, 32, 34, 95
  see also cheese; yoghurt
dehydration 42
detoxing 37, 40, 71–2
DHA fats 31, 46
diabetes 9, 11, 24
diaries 33
dill: Cucumber, Grape & Dill Salad 114
dinner planner, Phase 2 103
DNA 27
dressings: Chimichurri Dressing 57
  Creamy Avocado Dressing 88
  Mustard Dressing 59, 162
drinks 22, 42, 65, 95, 99, 104
dumplings: Cabbage Leaf Gyozas 133

E

eating disorders 24

eating out 35–6
eggs 30, 31, 95, 97
  Asparagus, Courgette & Herb Frittata 126
  Baked Green Eggs 129
  Spinach & Mushroom Wraps 125
electrolytes 42, 72–4
emotions 41, 49
emulsifiers 20
en Papillote, Aromatic Baked Bass 184
energy levels 24, 33, 40, 94, 96
entertaining 35
EPA 31, 46
epigenetics 27
Epsom salts 70, 74
equipment 53, 75
exercise 22, 49, 96
eye problems 46

F

fasting 20, 22, 66
fat cells: brown fat 45
  fat burning 20, 94
  toxins stored in 37, 42
  white fat 45
fats, in diet 29, 31
feasting 20, 23
fennel: Braised Chicken with Fondant Leeks & Fennel 165
  Pistou Soup with Parmesan Crisps 174
  Rainbow Slaw with Creamy Avocado Dressing 88
fennel seeds: Italian Pork & Fennel Meatballs 168
Feta with Levantine Tabbouleh 208
fibre 29, 45, 46
fight or flight mode 22, 49, 96
filaggrin deficiency 46
fish 30, 31
  oily fish 46
  Phase 2 95, 97, 99
  see also cod, salmon etc
flatbreads 106, 178
flaxseeds 31

food diaries 33
Fragrant Stir-fried Steak 190
freezers 51
French Onion & Thyme Soup 81
fridges 51
Frittata: Asparagus, Courgette & Herb 126
fruit 22, 29, 65, 98
   see also apples, pears etc

G

gallstones 70
garlic: Ambrosial Garlic Braised Chickpeas 192
  the Best Chicken Bone Stock 62
  Cauliflower & Roasted Garlic Soup 82
  Classic Vegetable Stock 63
  Garlic Braised Hispi Cabbage 90
  Mustard Dressing 59
  Pistou 58
  Stir-fried Tofu, Pak Choi & Broccoli with Ginger & Garlic 194
  Sunshine Saffron Cauliflower Rice Pilau 86
genes 27
ginger: Butternut Squash, Turmeric & Ginger Soup 80
  Carrot & Ginger Muffins 128
  Stir-fried Tofu, Pak Choi & Broccoli with Ginger & Garlic 194
GLA 31
GLP-1 drugs 9, 10
GLP-1 hormone 9–10, 43
glucose 43
glycogen 72
glyphosate 37
goat dairy foods 32
Goulash, Smokie Veggie 176
grains 31, 34
grapes 106
  Cucumber, Grape & Dill Salad with Tzatziki 114
Greek Salad 117, 158
green beans 45
  Butternut Squash & Green Bean Curry 87
  Fragrant Stir-fried Steak 190
  Kedgeree 134
  Pistou Soup with Parmesan Crisps 174
  Smash Burgers with Fondant Onion 138
  Spring Chicken Casserole 144
green vegetables 45
Guacamole 136
gut microbiome 20, 25, 29, 49
Gyozas, Cabbage Leaf 133

H

haddock see smoked haddock
halibut 46
Halloumi, Strawberry & Mint Salad 118
HBD Club 14, 17–18, 211
HBD Reset heroes 42–9
herbicides 37
herbs 45
  Chimichurri Dressing 57
  see also basil, thyme etc
herrings 46
high blood pressure 24, 48
Hippocrates 25
holidays 35–6
hormones 24
  fats and 31
  GLP-1 9–10
  stress hormones 22, 49, 96
hotels 36
Hummus, Lemon & Coriander 205
hunger 10, 38, 40, 49

I

immune system 20, 31, 38, 42
inflammation 10–11, 27, 30, 31
ingredients 42–8, 50–2
  Phase 1 68–9
  Phase 2 97–9
Institute for Optimal Nutrition (ION), London 17
insulin 9, 11, 20, 30, 43, 72

iron 29
Italian Pork & Fennel Meatballs 168

J

Jambalaya 139
joint pain 24
journalling 49

K

kale 45
Kedgeree 134
Ketchup, Red Pepper 56
kidneys 31, 70, 72
king prawns: King Prawn Paella 140
  Prawn & Mango Summer Rolls 198
kippers 46
Koftas, Lamb 149

L

lactose 32
lamb: Lamb Koftas with Baba Ganoush 149
  Moroccan Lamb Casserole with Squash & Spinach 172
  Moussaka 145
laxatives 70
leeks: Aromatic Baked Bass en Papillote 184
  Baked Green Eggs 129
  the Best Chicken Bone Stock 62
  Braised Chicken with Fondant Leeks & Fennel 165
  Classic Vegetable Stock 63
  Kedgeree 134
legumes 31
lemon: Lemon & Coriander Hummus with Crudites 205
  Lemon & Rosemary Monkfish Skewers 182
lemongrass: Chicken Satay Sliders with Creamy Avocado 202
  Thai-style Ramen 78
lentil rice 105

Jambalaya 139
lentils 30, 31
  Lentil Ragu with Rice 193
lettuce: Baba Ganoush 149
  Chicken Satay Sliders 202
  Chilli Beef Tacos 160
  Crispy Fish Tacos 136
  Prawn & Mango Summer Rolls 198
  Shredded Chicken & Tarragon Salad 120
  Tricolore Wrap 206
Levantine Tabbouleh 208
lifestyle diseases 11
liver disease 45
lunch planner, Phase 2 103

M

mackerel 31, 46
  see also smoked mackerel
magnesium 29, 30, 45, 70, 72, 74
main meal planner, Phase 2 103
malic acid 43
mangoes: Mango Chutney 61
  Mango Salsa 154
  Prawn & Mango Summer Rolls 198
  Sweet & Sour Salmon 156
meat 30, 31
  Phase 2 95, 97
  see also beef, lamb etc
meatballs: Italian Pork & Fennel Meatballs 168
  Steaming Hungarian Meatball Broth 170
Mediterranean diet 13, 22, 23
metabolism 14, 41, 48
microbiome, gut 20, 25, 29, 49
midlife changes 20
migraines 24
milk 104
minerals 29–30, 45, 72–4
mint: Halloumi, Strawberry & Mint Salad 118
monkfish: Lemon & Rosemary Monkfish Skewers 182
monounsaturated fats 46

mood 24
Moroccan Lamb Casserole with
   Squash & Spinach 172
motivation 36–7
Moussaka 145
Muffins, Carrot & Ginger 128
muscles 48
mushrooms: Cabbage Leaf Gyozas 133
   Lentil Ragu with Rice 193
   Moussaka 145
   Shiitake Mushroom, Spinach & Thyme Risotto 142
   Spinach & Mushroom Wraps 125
   Thai-style Ramen 78
   Truffle Mushroom Tarts with Emmental 187
Mustard Dressing 59, 162

N

nervous system 22, 49
neurodegenerative diseases 38
nightshade vegetables 27, 32, 33, 34, 65, 68
non-scale victories (NSVs) 23
nori seaweed wrappers: Tuna Sushi 200
nuts 30, 31, 46, 48, 97
   see also walnuts

O

obesity 27
oils 31
oily fish 46
oleic acid 46
olive oil 23
olives: Caponata with Cod 153
   Greek Salad 15, 117
omega-3 fats 31, 46, 48
omega-6 fats 31
omnivores 22
onions: the Best Chicken Bone Stock 62
   Cauliflower & Roasted Garlic Soup 82
   Chana Masala with Flatbreads 178
   Chilli Beef Tacos 160
   Classic Beef Stew with Thyme 166
   Classic Vegetable Stock 63
   French Onion & Thyme Soup 81
   Garlic Braised Hispi Cabbage with Caramelised Onions 90
   Lentil Ragu with Rice 193
   Mango Salsa 154
   Smash Burgers with Fondant Onion 138
   Steaming Hungarian Meatball Broth 170
   Stir-fried Tofu, Pak Choi & Broccoli 194
   Tomato Carpaccio with Avocado, Red Onion & Basil 84
   see also shallots; spring onions
oral allergy syndrome 45
oyster mushrooms: Spinach & Mushroom Wraps 125

P

Paella, King Prawn 140
pain 24
pak choi: Aromatic Baked Bass en Papillote 184
   Fragrant Stir-fried Steak 190
   Stir-fried Tofu, Pak Choi & Broccoli 194
   Thai-style Ramen 78
pans 53
pantry ingredients 50
parasympathetic nervous system 49, 96
Parmesan Crisps 174
parsley: Chimichurri Dressing 57
pasta 105
Pate, Smoked Mackerel 204
patties: Lamb Koftas with Baba Ganoush 149
pears: Waldorf Salad 112
peas 30, 45
pectin 45
Pennebaker, James 49
peppers 27, 33
   Baked Feta Parcels 150
   Caponata with Cod 153
   Feta with Levantine Tabbouleh 208
   Greek Salad 117, 158

Italian Pork & Fennel Meatballs 168
Jambalaya 139
King Prawn Paella 140
Mango Salsa 154
Red Pepper Ketchup 56
Smokie Veggie Goulash 176
Sweet & Sour Salmon 156
Tempeh Chilli with Cauliflower Rice 177
Tricolore Wrap 206
pesticides 37
Phase 1 13–14, 21, 34, 65–75
  checklist 75
  detoxing 71–4
  Epsom salts 70
  food list 68–9
  Lizzie's HBD tips 67, 71
  preparation 65–6
  soups and main meals 77–91
  withdrawal symptoms 71
Phase 2 13–14, 21, 93–107
  breakfasts 102, 109–29
  food list 97–9
  Lizzie's HBD tips 94–5, 105–6
  main meal planner 103
  a perfect HBD Phase 2 day 100
  rules 96
  treats 106
Phase 3 14, 21, 23, 210
Phase 4 21, 23, 210
Pilaf, Chicken Cauliflower Rice 186
Pilau, Sunshine Saffron Cauliflower Rice 86
Pistou 58
  Pistou Soup with Parmesan Crisps 174
Pizza, Cauliflower 188
plant protein 48
polyphenols 29, 45
pomegranate seeds: Chicken & Pomegranate Tagine 152
  Pomegranate Couscous 146
pork: Cabbage Leaf Gyozas 133
  Italian Pork & Fennel Meatballs 168
  Steaming Hungarian Meatball Broth 170

portion sizes 34
potassium 46, 72
poultry 30, 97
  see also chicken
prawns: King Prawn Paella 140
  Prawn & Mango Summer Rolls 198
preservatives 20
problematic foods 32–3
protein 22, 29, 30–1, 48, 97
pulses 30, 97
pumpkin: Apple & Pumpkin Spiced Crumble Pots 122
puréeing stews 105

Q
quinoa 30–1

R
radishes: Crab Sliders 197
  Pomegranate Couscous 146
  Quick Pickles 204
  Scandi Mackerel Salad 162
  Waldorf Salad 112
Ragu, Lentil 193
rainbow chard: Smoked Haddock & Wilted Greens 121
Rainbow Slaw with Creamy Avocado Dressing 88
Ramen, Thai-style 78
red cabbage: Breakfast Slaw 110
  Crispy Fish Tacos 136
  Rainbow Slaw 88
  Tuna Sushi 200
  see also cabbage
Red Pepper Ketchup 56
reducing method, stews 105
respiratory tract infections 17
rest 37–8, 40
restaurants 36
rice see cauliflower rice; chickpea rice; lentil rice
risotto 105

Butternut Squash & Sage Risotto 171
Shiitake Mushroom, Spinach & Thyme Risotto 142
rocket: Avocado & Smoked Salmon Salad 113
Halloumi, Strawberry & Mint Salad 118
Shredded Chicken & Tarragon Salad 120
Tricolore Wrap 206
Truffle Mushroom Tarts with Emmental 187
root vegetables 30
see also carrots
Roper, Debbie 18
rye bread 23, 30

S

saffron: King Prawn Paella 140
Saffron Couscous 152
Sunshine Saffron Cauliflower Rice Pilau 86
sage: Butternut Squash & Sage Risotto 171
salads 45
Avocado & Smoked Salmon Salad 113
Caponata with Cod 153
Cucumber, Grape & Dill Salad with Tzatziki 114
Greek Salad 117, 158
Halloumi, Strawberry & Mint Salad 118
Scandi Mackerel Salad 162
Shredded Chicken & Tarragon Salad 120
Waldorf Salad 112
see also slaw
salmon 31, 46
Sweet & Sour Salmon 156
see also smoked salmon
Salsa, Mango 154
sardines 31, 46
Sarno, John 49
sauces: Curry Sauce 60
Red Pepper Ketchup 56
Scandi Mackerel Salad 162
sea bass 46
Aromatic Baked Bass en Papillote 184
Crispy Fish Tacos with Spicy Guacamole 136
Crispy Sea Bass with Mango Salsa 154
sea bream: Baked Sea Bream with
Mash & Greens 181
seafood 97
seasonings 99
seeds 30, 31, 46, 95, 97
shallots: Ambrosial Garlic Braised Chickpeas 192
Shawarma, Chicken 158
sheep dairy foods 32
shellfish 31
shiitake mushrooms: Shiitake Mushroom, Spinach & Thyme Risotto 142
Thai-style Ramen 78
Shredded Chicken & Tarragon Salad 120
skewers: Chicken Satay Sliders 202
Lemon & Rosemary Monkfish Skewers 182
skin 24, 46
slaw: Breakfast Slaw 110
Rainbow Slaw with Creamy Avocado Dressing 88
see also salads
sleep 24, 38, 40, 74
Sliders: Chicken Satay Sliders 202
Crab Sliders 197
slimming drugs 9
Smash Burgers with Fondant Onion 138
smoked haddock: Kedgeree 134
Smoked Haddock & Wilted Greens 121
smoked mackerel: Scandi Mackerel Salad 162
Smoked Mackerel Pate with Quick Pickles 204
Smoked Mackerel Sushi 116
smoked salmon: Avocado & Smoked Salmon Salad 113
Smokie Veggie Goulash 176
Smoky Tofu Hash 124
socca breads 106
sodium 72
soups: Butternut Squash, Turmeric & Ginger Soup 80
Cauliflower & Roasted Garlic Soup 82
French Onion & Thyme Soup 81
Pistou Soup with Parmesan Crisps 174
Steaming Hungarian Meatball Broth 170
Thai-style Ramen 78
soy 30, 48, 97

spices 33
Spicy Guacamole 136
spinach: Butternut Squash & Sage Risotto 171
   Chana Masala with Flatbreads 178
   Moroccan Lamb Casserole with Squash & Spinach 172
   Shiitake Mushroom, Spinach & Thyme Risotto 142
   Spinach & Mushroom Wraps 125
   Truffle Mushroom Tarts with Emmental 187
Spring Chicken Casserole 144
spring greens: Baked Sea Bream with Mash & Greens 181
   Spring Chicken Casserole 144
spring onions: Asparagus, Courgette & Herb Frittata 126
   Shredded Chicken & Tarragon Salad 120
   Smoked Haddock & Wilted Greens 121
   Smoked Mackerel Sushi 116
Springsteen, Bruce 41
squash see butternut squash
starches 29
Steak, Fragrant Stir-fried 190
Steaming Hungarian Meatball Broth 170
stews and casseroles 105
   Chicken & Pomegranate Tagine 152
   Classic Beef Stew with Thyme 166
   Moroccan Lamb Casserole 172
   Smokie Veggie Goulash 176
   Spring Chicken Casserole 144
   Tempeh Chilli with Cauliflower Rice 177
Stir-fried Tofu, Pak Choi & Broccoli with Ginger & Garlic 194
stocks 50, 65, 99
   the Best Chicken Bone Stock 62
   Classic Vegetable Stock 63
stomach acid 49
strawberries: Halloumi, Strawberry & Mint Salad 118
stress hormones 22, 49, 96
sugar burning 94
sugars 29–30
Summer Rolls, Prawn & Mango 198
Sunshine Saffron Cauliflower Rice Pilau 86
sushi: Smoked Mackerel Sushi 116
   Tuna Sushi 200
Sweet & Sour Salmon 156
sweet potatoes 28, 30
Swiss chard: Smoky Tofu Hash 124
sympathetic nervous system 22, 49, 96
symptoms, Phase 1 71–2

T

Tabbouleh, Levantine 208
tacos: Chilli Beef Tacos 160
   Crispy Fish Tacos with Spicy Guacamole 136
Tagine, Chicken & Pomegranate 152
tamari: Stir-fried Tofu, Pak Choi & Broccoli 194
   Tuna Sushi 200
tarragon: Shredded Chicken & Tarragon Salad 120
tarts: Truffle Mushroom Tarts with Emmental 187
tea 22, 42, 65, 99, 104
tempeh 48
   Tempeh Chilli with Cauliflower Rice 177
Thai-style Ramen 78
thirst 42
thyme: Classic Beef Stew with Thyme 166
   French Onion & Thyme Soup 81
   Shiitake Mushroom, Spinach & Thyme Risotto 142
tofu 48
   Smoky Tofu Hash 124
   Stir-fried Tofu, Pak Choi & Broccoli 194
tomatoes 27, 33
   Butternut Squash & Green Bean Curry 87
   Chana Masala with Flatbreads 178
   Feta with Levantine Tabbouleh 208
   Greek Salad 117, 158
   Jambalaya 139
   Mango Salsa 154
   Pistou Soup with Parmesan Crisps 174
   Pomegranate Couscous 146
   Tomato Carpaccio with Avocado, Red Onion & Basil 84
   Tricolore Wrap 206
toxins 37, 42

travel 36
treats 20, 23, 106
Tricolore Wrap 206
Truffle Mushroom Tarts with Emmental 187
Tuna Sushi 200
turbot 46
turmeric: Butternut Squash, Turmeric & Ginger Soup 80
Tzatziki 114

U
ultra-processed foods (UPFs) 20, 24, 27, 37, 48
urea 31
ursolic acid 45

V
vegan diet 22, 30, 46
vegetables 22, 29, 33, 45
　Classic Vegetable Stock 63
　Phase 1 65, 68
　Phase 2 98
　see also carrots, tomatoes etc
vegetarian diet 22, 31
vinegar see apple cider vinegar
vitamins 29–30
vitamin B complex 30
vitamin C 30

W
Waldorf Salad 112
walking 49
walnuts 31, 46, 48, 95
　activating 48
　Apple & Pumpkin Spiced Crumble Pots 122
　Breakfast Slaw 110
　Waldorf Salad 112
water, drinking 22, 42, 65
weekends 35
weight loss 10, 24, 30, 40
weights, food 104
Weller, Cath 22, 74
wheat 27, 106
white fat 45
wholefoods 22
wholegrains 30
wind 32
withdrawal symptoms 71–2
wraps: Spinach & Mushroom Wraps 125
　Tricolore Wrap 206

Y
yoghurt 32, 97
　Tzatziki 114

BE THE HEALTHIEST, LIGHTEST, HAPPIEST VERSION OF YOU, *FOR LIFE*

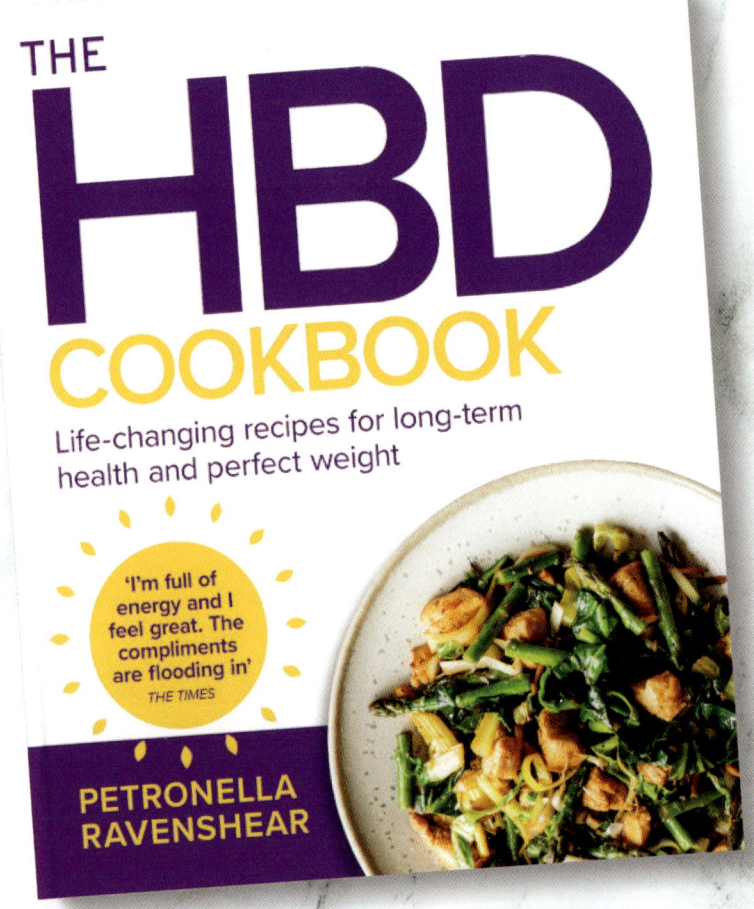

Continue your Human Being Diet journey, all year round, with a helping hand from *The HBD Cookbook*, out now.

A companion to *The Human Being Diet*, these easy and delicious recipes give you the perfect toolkit to help maintain your balanced metabolism and glowing health.

'I feel renewed. I'd battled my relationship with food for so many years and now I'm healthy and I feel fantastic. It's a feeling money can't buy'

HBD COMMUNITY MEMBER

Find out more: www.thehumanbeingdiet.com